THE AIDS DISASTER

The Failure of Organizations in New York and the Nation

Charles Perrow and Mauro F. Guillén

Yale University Press   New Haven and London

Set in Times Roman type by Marathon
Typography Service, Inc., Durham, North
Carolina.
Printed in the United States of America
by Vail-Ballou Press, Binghamton,
New York.

Library of Congress Cataloging-in-
Publication Data
Perrow, Charles.
The AIDS disaster : the failure of organ-
izations in New York and the nation /
Charles Perrow and Mauro F. Guillén.
    p.   cm.
Includes bibliographical references and
index.
ISBN 0-300-04879-3 (alk. paper).—
ISBN 0-300-04880-7 (pbk. : alk. paper)
1. AIDS (Disease)—New York. 2. AIDS
(Disease)—Social aspects—United
States. I. Guillén, Mauro F. II. Title.
RA644.A25P45 1990
362.1'969792'0097471—dc20
90-37170 CIP

The paper in this book meets the guidelines
for permanence and durability of the
Committee on Production Guidelines for
Book Longevity of the Council on Library
Resources.

10 9 8 7 6 5 4 3 2 1

To those who died young

CONTENTS

ACKNOWLEDGMENTS

The American Foundation for AIDS Research (AmFAR) funded the first part of this project, which consisted of interviews with about sixty public and private organizations or subunits of organizations in New York City. AmFAR took a risk in doing so. The principal investigator had not worked in the health field for twenty years, and he posed an unconventional question: whether organizational theory could contribute to understanding the dynamics of the AIDS epidemic.

Our thanks are due to the many people in New York City whom we interviewed and to the organizations that gave us access. Some did so with understandable reluctance, some respondents were very guarded, as we shall see, and some organizations found it necessary to deny interviews. We believe that Chapter 8 will explain why. But there were other respondents who were performing heroic tasks in hostile and beggarly environments and doing work of such importance that we can only be immensely grateful for the time they gave us.

Although our interviews helped us conceptualize the problem, the interview data are not the main focus of this book, which relies primarily on published materials. We needed to put the behavior of organizations in New York City into a larger perspective, and here the remarkable book by Randy Shilts, *And the Band Played On*, was invaluable for understanding the early years. Intertwined with dramatic reconstructions of personal lives was a well-documented, month-by-month account of the failure of key organizations at the national level to intervene in a meaningful way in what was fast becoming a problem of disastrous proportions.

Shilts wrote at a time when the focus of many was primarily on male homosexuals; our own interviews and, increasingly, health officials and the daily press drew attention to AIDS among drug users and among inner-city blacks and Hispanics. Inevitably, this new information drew us into social issues that reached beyond the gay community and the initial failure of federal, state, and local organizations to provide for education and care. We increasingly relied on newspaper accounts as it became more and more obvious that poverty, homelessness, syphilis, discrimination, intravenous injection of drugs, and finally crack cocaine would be the context for what could be called the second epidemic. We want to thank especially the many journalists writing for the *New York Times* in this connection and, among public health researchers, Samuel Friedman and his co-workers at The Narcotic and Drug Research, Inc.

The Institution for Social and Policy Studies at Yale University, Joseph LaPalombara, director, gave us much valuable help over the three years that the project has run, most notably the services of an extraordinary secretary who became in effect the very resourceful project administrator, Barbara Boggs. Melinda Cuthbert organized the first wave of interviews and provided an invaluable perspective in the first year of the project. Mauro Guillén, a Ph.D. candidate in the Department of Sociology at Yale University, joined the project in its second year as an interviewer and soon became a collaborator with the principal investigator.

The intellectual commentaries our work has received have been extraordinary; we know we have not answered all criticisms, but our attempts to do so have greatly improved the final product. The following list of names is assuredly incomplete: Rikki Abzug, Lee Clarke, Paul DiMaggio, Sam Friedman, Eliot Freidson, Nick Grouf, Peter D. Hall, Edward Kaplan, Mathilde Krim, Philip Leaf, Bernd Marin, Asbjorn Osland, Donald Palmer, Edith Perrow, George Silver, Sim Sitkins, Rosemary Taylor, David Tobis, and Robert Zussman. Finally, we applaud the editorial courage of Gladys Topkis.

1 INTRODUCTION

In what may prove to be the quintessential comment on New York City's reaction to the AIDS crisis of some eight years' duration, the *New York Times* of March 7, 1989, headlined its Metropolitan News section: "AIDS Drives Jobs Away, Study Shows. Jammed Hospitals Raise Specter of 'a Calcutta.'" AIDS, the cynic might observe, will arouse the city's powerful to action only when it drives away business and interferes with the ability of the well-to-do to receive emergency medical care at their hospitals. Only then will the mayor be moved to action, as Mayor Koch was two months later, when he announced a more substantial response than several previous announced responses to warnings from less prestigious sources.

The study the *Times* reported was financed by several large foundations, and the meeting to discuss it was attended by elite businessmen. The study warned that "businesses—facing a city gripped by plague-like conditions in subways, terminals and streets—will leave for a less daunting environment." The chairman of Time, Inc., a member of the group, was quoted as saying, "When the world realizes New York has not got any empty hospital beds, people will think twice about moving here. It's a frightening thought."[1]

1. Lambert, "AIDS Drives Jobs Away." Full citations for works mentioned by authors and short titles in the footnotes are given in the Bibliography.

Frightening as it is, it is hardly a new thought, and the crisis that is trivialized by reference to bed shortages for non-AIDS patients was amply heralded and need not have been nearly as severe. Ultimately, economic elites and political elites—symbolized in this story by Time's chairman, Mayor Koch, Governor Cuomo, and then-President Reagan—could fairly be charged with the responsibility. But in greater measure the failure of New York City, New York State, and the federal government to cope with the AIDS crisis has a more prosaic source. It is in considerable part a story of organizational failures at the local, state, and national levels. Specific organizations—run by people of average competence and charged with carrying out a variety of tasks from education to health care—failed, on what we believe is an unprecedented level, to do their jobs.

For example, the city and the state (and the federal government) were warned years ago about the broad dimensions of a crisis that would include, but go far beyond, a shortage of hospital beds; yet the city was still closing down hospital beds as late as 1987. The epidemic was identified in 1981; but New York City did not begin funding for AIDS until well into 1984, when there were already 1,700 cases. The federal government refused to spend funds appropriated by Congress throughout the 1980s, even delaying screening of the blood supply for budgetary reasons and thus continuing the spread of the virus among transfusion recipients. Governor Cuomo of New York State more than once refused to spend money that the state legislature had appropriated. A government study released in June 1989 argued that the Centers for Disease Control had underestimated by one-third the number of people in the United States infected with the virus.[2] Dr. C. Everett Koop, the Surgeon General, was quoted in 1988 as saying, "How many are infected? . . . We use the number of a million or a million and a half, but it could be 400,000 or it could be 4 million. We just don't know."[3]

Why has it taken a threat to business opportunities to elicit the concern of the city's elites? Why was there not an appropriate response

2. "Forecasts of AIDS Fall Short."
3. Lambert, "Puzzling Questions Are Raised on Statistics."

seven or even five or three years ago? That is the subject of this book. Three "layers" of explanation will be considered. The first is the layer of "proximate causes": homophobia, discrimination, politics and ideology, and a generally failing health care sector.

But beyond this lies a more pervasive explanation: the AIDS epidemic itself is sufficiently distinctive to hamper the ability of organizations to respond according to their mandates. This second layer, the "organizational" level of explanation, argues that the proximate causes might have been overcome if organizations had carried out their mandates to a reasonable degree. The performance of organizations seems unusually poor, so poor as to suggest that there is something special about this crisis. AIDS, we will argue, differs strikingly from other epidemics and public health crises in three ways: because the cost is so high, because the possibility of unsuspected transmission provokes an unusual degree of fear (for death appeared certain), and because the disease is so strongly associated with stigmatized groups — gay men and intravenous drug users (IVDUs).

If AIDS is unique as a public health problem, does that mean that we could not be expected to have handled it any better? We will argue against this position. The essentials of the disease — that it is a blood-borne virus infecting men and women, straights as well as gays, and that it is responsive to ridiculously cheap prevention measures (bleach and condoms) — were all known in the first year, yet no education or warning campaign was mounted, nor was blood tested or the donors screened. Understanding why there was such a widespread failure to respond is the central task of this book.

The third "layer" of explanation will concern us as we narrow in on New York City, where one-fifth of the national cases are concentrated and most of our research was done. It is not often that we find a problem that so draws upon, sucks in, and is magnified by so many other problems. The essence of the mishandling of the AIDS crisis is ultimately not an organizational failure so much as the failure of society to overcome poverty and discrimination. AIDS came along at just the wrong time: the 1970s and 1980s witnessed an upheaval in sexual norms, a growing underclass, and an ethic based upon free-market assumptions about maximizing individual self-interest. AIDS, and the consequences of these social changes, will be with us for a long time. We hope that our study will put them into some perspective and prepare us for "the loss of jobs because of the bed shortage" that will be the most trivial of the tragedies.

As the AIDS epidemic continues its course, it becomes more and more necessary to tell the tale of organizational failure, because we have a strong, Orwellian tendency to forget and to revise the past. As 1982, 1983, and 1984 recede, we forget how clear the warnings were, how strong the evidence was, and how deliberately public officials and private groups failed to respond. Attempts to revise that dismal record, through outright lies and convenient excuses, will only leave us less prepared to cope with new phases of the AIDS epidemic—in the 1990s AIDS will more and more be seen as a disease of the ghetto—and with new epidemics that may be impending. (Possible mutations of the AIDS virus that make it hardier and more easily transmitted are unlikely, but not inconceivable.) As the world becomes more tightly integrated with easy foreign travel and large migrations of refugees, we may see new epidemics appearing.

Our thesis is that the proximate causes of ideology and politics do not sufficiently explain the organizational and institutional failures; an additional explanation, one based on the particular characteristics of AIDS, is required. AIDS is unique among epidemics in the United States in its ability to disable organizational and community defenses and in its interaction with the pervasive social problems of poverty and discrimination.

We can foresee three possible reactions to our thesis, although there might be more. One is that widespread homophobia and racism are sufficient explanations; organizational failures merely reflect these attitudes and practices and were to be expected. The second denies that there is anything to explain since there has not been a massive failure to respond but an adequate, even quite good response. This tends to be the position of many, though not all, government and scientific spokesmen. The third, the cynical response, also denies that there is anything to explain, this time because one should not expect anything better from the American health care sector. History discloses that it has always been thus, that the failure is similar to failures in most systems or in organizations in general. In this view, to assert the presence of unique characteristics is both wrong and, worst of all, an invitation to indignation, which reportedly interferes with research.

We will take up the first of these reactions, that discrimination against gay men and minorities explains the failure, in this introductory chapter; the second—that there has been no failure—in Chapter 2; and the third —that we should expect failure—in Chapters 2 and 3. Chapter 4 presents the argument that AIDS is unique. Then, having argued that there is, indeed, something to explain and that homophobia and racism are insufficient, we shall move on to the experience of New York City to offer an organizational analysis and study the interaction of AIDS with poverty and neglect in Chapters 5 through 9. We focus on the period 1981–1988, for it was during these years that the organizational response took shape.

DISCRIMINATION AS AN EXPLANATION
FOR RESPONSE FAILURE

It is important to discuss at the outset the explanation based on hostility toward gay men, since we find it insufficient. Our stance involves quite controversial matters, and we should make our position clear. At present the largest number of AIDS cases are males who are homosexual or bisexual. Society by and large rejects these forms of sexual behavior, and the feelings underlying this rejection could cause organizations that would otherwise care for the sick or educate the healthy about prevention to fail to do even a minimally adequate job. (Note that while the term *homophobia* is often used to describe hostility toward those with a sexual preference for someone of the same gender, it originally meant something more specific—a fear that one's own latent homosexuality will be expressed. Hostility toward homosexuals presumably includes more than that fear.)

It is easy to make the case that society has been slow to respond because of the behavior of gay men. Sexual transmission of the disease appears to happen most effectively in anal intercourse, with the receptor being vulnerable because of the tearing of tissue in the anus. The trauma of anal penetration causes bleeding, and the blood comes in contact with the semen, which contains the virus. Gay men engaging in frequent anal intercourse have always been susceptible to diseases that can be spread through semen and blood, and a highly active homosexual male is very likely to have hepatitis B, a debilitating disease that can be treated but not cured, and to have had syphilis, gonorrhea, and other (nonfatal) sexually transmitted diseases. Anal intercourse is practiced by heterosexuals as well, but it is not a characteristic or principal form of sexual behavior and is presumably quite infrequent in this group as compared with its frequency in segments of the gay male population.

Given an uncommon sexual practice, frequently engaged in, and often with casual or anonymous partners, it is not surprising that many heterosexual citizens consider the disease self-inflicted and the product of "immoral," "unnatural," "repugnant" behavior. Given the many accounts of several impersonal sexual encounters at the "bathhouses," we can add the self-indulgent pursuit of risky behavior to the characterization of the gay population. This is an unfair characterization. Only a small percentage of gay men are believed to be highly promiscuous, perhaps not a significantly higher percentage of promiscuous behavior than can be found among young male heterosexuals. Still, the small numbers existed, and they were concentrated in cities such as San Francisco and New York, thus aiding the rapid spread of the disease.

Many gay groups initially fought to prevent the closing of bathhouses, even though public officials argued that they were a major disseminating mechanism. Their opposition to such public health measures added to the negative characterization of gay men and their groups. Finally, it might be thought that if a cure or vaccine for AIDS were found, at great public expense, the offending behavior would once again be carried on by large numbers of gay men and the bathhouses would open again. AIDS would be like syphilis, treatable and thus worth a risk. (The sexual transmission of the disease in the United States appears to be primarily via anal sex; it was thought—though with increasingly less certainty—to be spread by mouth-to-genital contact, mouth-to-anus contact, called "rimming," and contact with urine, called "golden showers."[4]

4. Winkelstein et al., "Sexual Practices and Risk of Infection."

None of these practices is likely to win acceptance from the general population, though mouth-to-genital contact is surely practiced by many heterosexuals.) Given these paths of transmission, the widespread rejection of homosexuality in the population even before the AIDS epidemic, and the exaggerated estimates of promiscuity, it is reasonable to assume that rejection of homosexuality and even fear of it (homophobia) have shaped the public response to AIDS.

Similarly, intravenous drug use is shunned by the majority of Americans. The behavior is seen as self-indulgent, and AIDS transmitted in this way is seen as self-inflicted, especially since the use of sterilized needles would prevent transmission. In this view, if needles and syringes that were self-cleaning or not reusable were made available, or if the dealers were to protect their customers by enclosing, with each packet of heroin, a sterile needle and syringe, a cup for heating, and cotton for straining, the offending behavior would just continue.

In this fashion the AIDS epidemic has become "moralized" far more than "medicalized." In the countries of continental Europe, in contrast, the existence of integrated health systems has made a medicalized response to the disease possible from the outset. In Europe health professionals have much more control over the definition of the disease than in the United States, and they have emphasized the biological rather than the social aspects. Drug users, for example, are viewed not as self-indulgent and self-destructive individuals but as persons with a biochemical problem that requires physiological and psychological treatment. This has allowed education campaigns to take place, prevented widespread discrimination, and encouraged the development of hospices and other places of treatment. For example, a public school in Austria that tried to exclude a young child who was HIV-positive (and thus would be expected to develop the symptoms of AIDS eventually) was summarily prevented from barring the child by the top educational official in the government, and his action was announced on national television.[5] In contrast, the saga of a Florida family with an HIV-positive child went on for months,

5. We are grateful to Bernd Marin of the European Centre in Vienna for the distinction between moralizing and medicalizing, for alerting us to this last incident,

and the debate about allowing such children to attend schools here has been protracted.

In addition to the moralizing definition of AIDS in the United States, a definition that conjures up images of pollution and degeneracy,[6] we have racial stigmatization to deal with. Drug users with AIDS are disproportionately black or Hispanic, and minorities will soon constitute the largest percentage of AIDS cases in the United States. Concern with the health or general well-being of these minority groups has never been high in America. Black convicts were subjected to ghoulish and inhuman experiments as recently as the 1950s.[7] Access to health care, and thus presumably concern about health, has always been minimal for impoverished groups and especially for the minorities among them.

One of the consequences of the public's rejection of homosexuality and drug use, and their presumed seductiveness, is that some spokespersons (even in the black community) have taken the stand that *it is better to let the guilty die of AIDS than to risk encouraging extramarital sex or drug abuse among the still innocent.* In this view, which makes it nearly impossible to mount education campaigns, encouraging homosexual men to use condoms or drug users to use sterilized "works" condones their acts; furthermore, it would be wrong if the education campaigns convinced "innocent" people to try either homosexuality or intravenous drugs.

Thus, much of the failure to fund education campaigns and even care and treatment programs must be laid to these attitudes, which are pre-

---

and for supplying informal information about AIDS in Europe. For a comparative study, see Fox, Day, and Klein, "The Power of Professionalism." The authors argue, mistakenly we believe, that AIDS public policy in all these countries "has, in the main, been based on consensus both professional and political" (p. 94). We would exclude the United States, and perhaps Britain, from this characterization.

6. Sontag, *AIDS and Its Metaphors.*

7. See Jones, *Bad Blood.* In 1932, the Public Health Service initiated a series of experiments in Alabama "that insured that some 400 Black sharecroppers would never be treated for their syphilitic infections." The experiments were reported in scholarly journals, as is customary in medical research, and did not end until the general press aired the issue in 1972 (Brandt, *No Magic Bullet,* pp. 158–159).

sumed to be widespread. (Public opinion polls show little sympathy for gay men, intravenous drug users, and their spouses.)[8]

In our view, hostility toward sexual and racial minorities in connection with the epidemic is not confined to the "moral majority" or religious fundamentalists, though it is outspoken among these groups. It is a common reaction in presumably more sophisticated circles, including academic and professional ones, though it is rarely explicit there. It emerges from some self-interested concerns that are not ideological but that quickly evoke or awaken the sexual and racial stigmas that no citizen born and raised in the United States can avoid.

For example, there is concern about the strain upon medical and social resources caused by the epidemic. Though none would speak for attribution, doctors and medical researchers we have talked with in New York City and at various universities say that many of their colleagues resent that their research funds and resources are being diverted to a "plague" that is self-inflicted; medical educators are concerned that their hospitals cannot attract the best interns and residents if medical students believe that the variety of patient disorders they will treat will be limited because of a large number of AIDS patients. Middle- and upper-class citizens fear that there will be no bed available when they have their heart attack or need an elaborate bypass or transplant operation. These concerns may provoke a prejudiced and homophobic reaction. A great many people in our society share these feelings; some are even willing to let people die in the streets, without succor or the dignity associated with normal human rights.

As sociologists, we do not find that the attitudes of the public toward drug abusers, minorities, and homosexuals fully explain the failure of organizations and public policy in general. "Fear and loathing" have played a major role, of course, but we have organizational mechanisms to protect minorities from these attitudes. Although the mechanisms are quite imperfect, they have some effect. Why so little effect in this case? Why did existing organizations fail, and why are so few new ones succeeding?

8. Kagay, "Poll Finds Antipathy towards AIDS Victims."

If intolerance were all that mattered, the repression of homosexuals and minorities would have been fiercer than it has been, and it would not have required the AIDS epidemic to increase it. We do not exterminate gay people or those addicted to powerful drugs in our society, nor do we place them in concentration camps for life, as a matter of public policy.[9] They are not by law denied health insurance, though their health risks are great. It is not a public policy to discharge them from all employment upon disclosure of their behavior. Discrimination certainly exists, but most of it is not officially sanctioned.

Furthermore, our public officials go to considerable lengths to reassure these groups and the public at large that everything possible is being done to meet their health needs in the AIDS crisis—surely an unnecessary effort if widespread intolerance were to blame. If there is some tolerance in society for marginal groups, then we must explain why it has not been sufficient to permit a bending of "mainstream" rules (as, for example, distribution of sterile needles in drug rehabilitation centers) for the benefit of public health. To put it more directly, why did organizations fail to cope with and neutralize the hostile attitudes that were preventing effective action once AIDS was on the scene? This was not the first time that blacks, Hispanics, and homosexuals required public and voluntary services from organizations supposedly serving the public interest. Why did they fail more than usual?

We hope that our book will provide some answers. AIDS will not be the last epidemic, nor the last to affect primarily poor and stigmatized groups. We could at least learn something from our experience with it so far.

9. Cuban public health officials quarantined 240 healthy HIV carriers in a "sanitorium," at a complex of houses near Havana airport. See "The War on AIDS," a letter by Columbia University professors Jeanne Smith and Sergio Piomelli, *New York Times*, January 22, 1989, section 4, p. 24.

2   THE ORGANIZATIONAL FAILURE

AIDS has had a dramatic, fast-moving history in the years since 1981, when it was first "officially" identified. It was first called a gay men's disease, despite initial evidence that it was also associated with intravenous drug use and could be transmitted to newborn babies. The organizational response was slow and fumbling. As we shall see, a core of researchers, physicians, and politicians who foresaw the present crisis repeatedly called in vain for far more resources and education. When governmental responses finally appeared, this early record of inaction was ignored and even rewritten. The predictions about the number of cases and the fatality rates were almost universally very short of the mark; even in 1989, eight years into an epidemic that has killed nearly 70,000 and infected from 1 to 1.5 million in the United States alone, new surveys and more careful examination of existing data reveal higher rates of death and infection than official sources acknowledge.

In addition to the problem of inadequate responses and unrealistic predictions, the "cultural" associations of the disease have changed rapidly. AIDS has gone from a gay male disease to one of poor minorities; the definition of "risky" behavior has grown from gay sex to drug abuse, and from intravenous drug abuse to use of smokable cocaine or "crack"; and now the press emphasizes heterosexual transmission in crack houses and the infection of children. In fact, about 2 percent of new cases are

now pediatric.[1] Finally, the specter of bed shortages and hospital crowding will probably be supplanted by resentment of the enormous costs
that will be incurred when drugs are used to treat patients over the course
of a lifetime.

Despite the expansion of the population affected, another rapid change
has been an increase in the segregation of the newly affected minority
population. The drug-abuse connection may have "redlined" the disease into a geographical area of the inner city where the vast majority of
respectable citizens do not stray. Only in the big cities, where the ghettos spill over into the entertainment, banking, and commercial districts,
is there any significant contact between the majority and the infected
minority. And the fear that the disease will spread to the greater part of
the general population who are not poor and of no other color but a grey
pink has receded, uneasily, despite the evidence from Africa, where
men and women of all classes are involved.

With increasing research and experimentation has come another important shift: though there is still no known cure or vaccine, and some years
are likely to pass before there is one, palliatives are appearing, and in a
few years AIDS may be a fully treatable disease. In the early years it was
believed, though it could not be proved, that all who test positive for the
Human Immunodeficiency Virus (HIV) would eventually develop the
various diseases labeled the Acquired Immune Deficiency Syndrome,
and all would then die within two years or less. We are beginning to see
therapies that may delay the onset of "full-blown AIDS" in those who
test positive but have no symptoms and prolong the lives of those who
do show symptoms of AIDS. As will be discussed in Chapter 9, in the
future it may be possible to control the disease, much as hypertension or
diabetes can be controlled, and the person, while forever infected, will
be able to live a normal span, though incurring the associated disabilities of constant medication and perhaps retaining the ability to infect
others.

What kind of social world will exist when this control is possible we

---

1. Centers for Disease Control, *HIV / AIDS Surveillance Report*, p. 8. See also
"Study Finds Antibodies for AIDS in 1 in 61 Babies."

are not in a position to say. The problems of insurance, discrimination, and infectivity will be difficult ones. The costs of controlling the symptoms may easily exceed the costs of the present (ineffective) therapies and care. AIDS affects young people. If treatment insured a normal life span, during which the patient could still infect others, forty more years of unprotected sex or needle sharing would certainly spread the epidemic. On the other hand, a population in treatment would be accessible for preventive education; while some might infect others, we suspect that few would and that the infection rate would gradually drop to near zero.[2]

Our inquiry does not extend to that possibility. In the years our study focuses on, 1981–1988, only one drug, azidothymidine (AZT), was available for those who suffered, and in its initial dosage it was a strong poison that had many side effects and could give only limited help for a limited time. During this period gay males and IVDUs were the principal carriers and sufferers; infant and pediatric AIDS was only beginning to assume significance. And it was largely a period where there was substantial fear by the public that AIDS might spread to nonpoor heterosexuals. That fear appears to have declined as the spread has concentrated in previously segregated minority communities. Although we do not discuss the possibility of heterosexual spread in this account of organizational failures, we would like to observe that there are a substantial number of IVDUs in the middle and upper classes and a substantial number of gay men who harbor or will harbor and spread the virus in these classes, that bisexuality is quite possibly more widespread than is commonly believed, especially among the young, and that anal and oral sex is hardly unknown among heterosexuals. The gay and drug population is not safely encapsulated in gay and minority ghettos by any means, and there are many routes to nonpoor heterosexuals.

We are mostly interested in the period when the major organizational

2. Becker and Joseph, "AIDS and Behavioral Change"; Office of Technology Assessment, *How Effective Is AIDS Education?*; Turner, Miller, and Moses, eds., *AIDS*, pp. 259–356; Institute of Medicine, *Confronting AIDS: Update 1988* (Washington, D.C.: National Academy Press, 1988), pp. 64–69.

response was formed, 1981 to 1988, and we will try to avoid using hindsight as we document this response. But it should be noted at the outset that just as the AIDS story is a fast-moving one, so is the reconstruction of that history. As will be discussed in chapter 4, we interviewed officials in a number of organizations in New York City. We were surprised to find respondents in our interviews distorting recent events. (We even had to excise portions of our first draft because two of those we interviewed, after seeing the draft, denied that they had said what was reported.) Moreover, some AIDS historians appear to be altering the record. In general, the position taken in these reconstructions is that the response of officials and organizations was prompt and adequate. A special issue of the highly respected journal *Scientific American* in October 1988 is typical. It has little to say about the politics of AIDS or the response of government but lauds the response of the scientific community. It treats the most detailed history of the epidemic, Randy Shilts's *And the Band Played On*, in scathing terms in a book review.[3]

Since we draw heavily upon the Shilts book, a word about our use of it is appropriate. Shilts is often very passionate and angry, and there are many criticisms of his work from all quarters. We have therefore tried to examine other views. We accept his interview material as fact and have verified his references where possible. For a journalistic, even novelistic

---

3. See Shilts, *And the Band Played On*; and Blattner, "A Novelistic History." Blattner, of the National Cancer Institute, is understandably particularly disturbed by Shilts's assertion that the scientific community fumbled the ball in the early years; he calls "utterly naive" Shilts's statement that the AIDS virus was not a particularly difficult virus to find, ridicules the notion that making Dr. Gallo of the National Cancer Institute and Dr. Montagnier of France "co-discoverers" of the virus was "the result of some sort of political compromise," and asserts that "never has so much been accomplished so quickly in response to such a complex disease process." "To be sure," he admits, "the issue of timely funding for research was a problem" (but he neglects to note that virtually every study has documented this fully), and finally he does concede that there was some "inertia" in the response, which he claims Shilts sees as prejudice.

On the scientific ease of the discovery, we are not qualified to comment, but on the other matters we share Shilts's view, as overheated and "simplistic" as it may be.

account, the book is unusually good in its citations to literature and other forms of documentation. We share the opinion of Gerald Oppenheimer, a historian of the epidemic, that Shilts has been able to extend and deepen the public records with his interviewing.[4]

EARLY KNOWLEDGE OF THE DIMENSIONS
OF THE CRISIS

We shall use June 1981, the date of the first Centers of Disease Control (CDC) report on the disease, as "time 0" in our account. Subsequently it was learned that there were unidentified cases in the United States in the late 1970s and in sub-Saharan Africa in 1959, but for purposes of tracking the response to an epidemic the date of first official notification is considered the starting point.

Though this was to be denied or minimized later on, the dimensions of the disease were known in the first year: if affected homosexual men, intravenous drug users, both whites and blacks, and it could be passed on by a mother to her unborn child. These characteristics would seem to indicate massive education programs about sexual practices that could spread diseases and about the dangers of using unsterilized needles, both matters with which public health officials were familiar because of infections such as hepatitis B among gay men and IVDUs. They would also seem to mandate screening of the blood supply and the education of female sex partners of bisexual men, IVDUs, and hemophiliacs. None of these steps was taken in the first few years of the epidemic.

The disease was initially identified as a "gay disease," a disease of male homosexuals, and the term GRID, for "gay-related immune deficiency," was proposed in 1982. Yet in July 1981, just one month into the epidemic (T-1), IVDUs who were not gay men were identified as having the disease. The percentage of IVDU patients always ran far behind that of gay men, but there were always some IVDUs in the statistics. This itself might have given cause for alarm and for education campaigns, regardless of their difficulty.

4. Oppenheimer, "In the Eye of the Storm," p. 293.

At T-6, six months into the epidemic, three black infants, children of heterosexual intravenous drug users, had the same rare pneumonia and T-cell patterns common to gay pneumonia victims. With only a few cases by this time, intravenous drug use was strongly suspected as a means of transmission; blood was implicated; and the pattern of infection among homosexual males suggested that the same forms of intercourse associated with hepatitis B and other sexually transmitted diseases, such as rectal gonorrhea, primarily but not exclusively a gay men's disease, could spread the virus. At this point the resistance to a broad definition of the disease started. A paper about the infection of infants through infected mothers, wives of IVDUs, was prepared for the American Academy of Pediatrics but was rejected; the CDC requested a six-month budget to work on the disease, but the request was turned down; and Larry Kramer, a gay activist in New York City, attempted in vain to warn the gay male community that some high-risk sexual practices should be curtailed and the bathhouses restricted.[5]

The signs of denial and resistance in the government, medical community, and gay male community at T-6 were to continue, as our account will demonstrate. Eventually the medical community and then the gay male community dealt more forthrightly with the disease, and only in 1987 did the federal administration, in the form of the Presidential Commission on the Human Immunodeficiency Virus Epidemic, finally recognize the seriousness of the problem, but most of its recommendations were not acted upon.[6] Initially ill-starred because of the controversy about the qualifications and conservative views of the appointees, followed by staff wrangling and departures and commissioner resignations, the commission became surprisingly vigorous; it warned that the inter-

5. Shilts, *And the Band Played On*, pp. 210, 277, 418.
6. The report emphasizes two facts: the importance of trying to prevent the spread of the disease to avoid having to deal with expensive health care and certain death, on the basis of comparative costs arguments; and the potential outbreak of the epidemic into the rest of the population owing to the increasing incidence of AIDS among IVDUs (p. 94). It also argues that a major failure in the funding response to the crisis was the belief that AIDS was limited to a well-organized, affluent segment of the population (*Report of the Presidential Commission*, p. 117).

action of AIDS with long-standing societal problems, such as intravenous drug addiction, poverty, and homelessness, would spell disaster. It also criticized rigidity in money allocation for research and the fragmentation and financial inadequacy of the nation's health sector.

It will be important to keep in mind that the commission's report, as well as reports from the Office of Technology Assessment (OTA), the Congressional Research Service, the New York State Comptroller, the General Accounting Office (GAO), and the Institute of Medicine (IOM), and other groups, all speak of substantial funding failures and failures to educate; some speak of damaging infighting within the government and of the damaging role of conservative political groups. This record, merely outlined in the next sections, is in danger of being ignored.

FUNDING FAILURES

It is hard to prove a "funding failure" because no one can say what an adequate level of funding would have been. However, numerous government reports and those of professional research societies such as the Institute of Medicine assert that funding was slow in coming and hardly adequate.[7] A better indication of failure would be evidence that those who were most knowledgeable about the disease were unable to get anywhere near the funds they requested. More powerful evidence would be that these frustrated experts were forced to deny that they had asked for more money. And finally the most powerful evidence of a funding failure would be that even after funds had been budgeted, they were deliberately not allocated. Evidence of each scenario is provided by Shilts and the *Congressional Quarterly*.

Funding for work on the disease in the federal health establishment, and even in state health departments and state and private universities,

7. For a sampling of reports of inadequacy, see *Report of the Presidential Commission*; Office of Technology Assessment, *Review of the Public Health Service's Response*; New York State Comptroller, "Projected Cost of the Treatment"; General Accounting Office, *AIDS Prevention*. For Congressional Research Service and Institute of Medicine conclusions, see Shilts, *And the Band Played On*, pp. 213–214 and 586–587.

was a severe problem from the beginning and was not relieved until about six or seven years into the epidemic. Researchers at the CDC, for example, had to cannibalize other projects for several years, even after appropriations started flowing, according to interviews conducted by Randy Shilts and memos published in the *Congressional Quarterly*. Each year Congress voted substantially larger budgets for research, education, and treatment in the AIDS area than the Reagan administration requested, and the administration sometimes failed to spend all the funds. For example, Congress earmarked $5.6 million dollars for AIDS activities in fiscal 1982 and $28.7 million in 1983; neither the president's budget proposal nor any Public Health Service (PHS) agency request for those two years allocated any money to AIDS. In 1984, Congress obligated $61.5 million to AIDS (54 percent more than the president's request) and $97.4 million the following year (61 percent more).[8] More telling, Congress had to resort to the threat of legal action to get the data to confirm the widespread suspicion that officials were lying about the extent of their requests. Congress found that even as officials in the CDC, the National Cancer Institute (NCI), and other health agencies were testifying that they had all the funds they could wisely spend, they had been writing strong memos to their bosses pleading for more funds to meet the seriousness of the problem.

Despite Shilts's documentation of this serious charge, the other principal historian of AIDS (as of 1988), Sandra Panem, in *The AIDS Bureaucracy*, accepts the administration's denials that more money was needed.[9] In one dramatic episode, CDC Director William Foege asked a congressional staffer, Susan Steinmetz, to leave his office when she insisted on examining agency files regarding AIDS. Foege had claimed in speeches that there was no discrepancy between his requests for funds and his real needs. When Congress tried to verify this by sending Steinmetz to see him and his evidence, he argued that since the files contained the names of persons with AIDS, they were confidential. Con-

8. Office of Technology Assessment, *Review of the Public Health Service's Response*, p. 32.

9. Shilts, *And the Band Played On*; Panem, *The AIDS Bureaucracy*.

gress argued that they were looking not for names but for unfulfilled budget requests. Panem sides with Foege, whom she describes as a "religious man" with "steely acumen," driven to the uncharacteristic action of insisting that Steinmetz leave as "a measure of last resort," rather than Steinmetz, described as "stylish and energetic with a no-nonsense, aggressive approach to her work."

Randy Shilts, however, documents the charges of deception.[10] That same month, Foege had written a memo pleading for more funds and even attached fourteen pages listing studies that needed to be done and could be implemented if the needed funding was supplied. He was a consistent supporter of a more aggressive federal policy, though not publicly. One suspects he was ordered by his superiors to deny Steinmetz access to the records, including his own memos.

One of the authorities Panem quotes for the view that the health agencies had all the money they needed is Edward Brandt, assistant secretary for health, but Shilts quotes from an internal memo Brandt wrote in 1983 pleading for more money. In the memo Brandt also details the consequences for other programs of taking money from them for AIDS. Brandt desperately needed money. Shilts quotes from another Brandt memo to a House subcommittee asking for permission to transfer up to $12 million from the Health and Human Services Agency to AIDS activity—a significant increase at a time when the total budget for AIDS was only $28.7 million. Congress, as was its wont and as we can assume Brandt would predict, immediately authorized $12 million in *new* money. Finally, Congressman Silvio Conte inserted much of the material on the deception into the *Congressional Record* for May 25, 1983, so it was all available.[11]

10. Shilts, *And the Band Played On*, pp. 288–298.

11. *Congressional Record*, May 25, 1983, pp. H3341–3344. The discussion at that early date in the epidemic makes it clear that legislators were fully aware of both the alarming rate of new cases (doubling every six months), a gestation period of at least two years (the largest estimate they could have then; it has increased steadily and in 1989 was variously eight or ten years), and the impact upon the IVDU population. Even so, New York State and City officials argued that no one knew the epidemic would be so severe and not be limited to homosexual males.

The matter is important for three reasons. First, the record on AIDS is in danger of endorsing either the self-serving accounts of officials, as in Panem's book, or charges of homophobia on the part of government as a whole. Denis Altman's *AIDS in the Mind of America*,[12] for example, tends to blame the federal failure on massive homophobia, but the funding record establishes the pressures that agency heads such as Foege and Brandt, who wanted to do more, felt from the White House to hold back spending and spending requests. It also shows that Congress was more willing than the administration to fund programs. "Government," then, was not of one piece.

Second, the deceptions involving funding were still going on in 1988 and may continue into President Bush's administration. As late as July 1988, Senator Edward Kennedy was charging that federal officials were being forced by the White House to say all was fine when privately they knew it wasn't. In this case the charge concerned Dr. Anthony Fauci, the federal official in charge of testing AIDS drugs at the National Institute of Allergy and Infectious Diseases. There was, as one reporter put it, "an air of suspicion that Dr. Fauci was being compelled to defend the administration's policies rather than say what he believed." Fauci had admitted the previous April that it had taken an "inordinate time" to start trials on a promising drug, dextran sulfate, but he cited staff shortages and other mitigating circumstances. The test was designated a high priority in November, but approval for trials was not given until July.[13]

12. Denis Altman, *AIDS in the Mind of America*.
13. National Public Radio, "All Things Considered," July 24, 1988; and Boffey, "Tests of a Potential Drug." As the story of dextran sulfate shows, however, nothing is simple with AIDS. Gay activists claimed that a promising drug was being denied to them, but at least some researchers at the Federal Drug Administration suspected a problem: it was difficult, perhaps impossible, to absorb dextran sulfate into the bloodstream when it was administered orally. Yet, under pressure, clinical trials were finally set up. After some time it was announced that the trials were a disappointment; the drug was not absorbed from the gut into the blood, a problem that could have been identified by proper testing, using animals. Critics of the failure to conduct animal tests first insist that this is not an isolated instance; useless drugs are being administered to humans, they say. See the illuminating account of the drug industry and AIDS in Mahar, "Pitiless Scourge."

The impact of the fiscal restraint was severe. Research was delayed for the lack of trifling sums for key equipment; even a request for a basic textbook on retroviruses, the group that includes HIV, costing $150, had to be turned down by the CDC, according to Shilts's respondents. Arguments for new laboratories went unheeded. At the state level there was, of course, less research, but requests for funds for education and treatment were turned down almost everywhere, notably in New York and Massachusetts. Only in California, initially only in San Francisco, was there a reasonably adequate response.[14] The inadequacy of funding in the nation was not due to a lack of vigorous warnings; there were impressive statistics and strong arguments that investment in research and prevention would forestall massive bills later. The dimensions of the crisis were seen as enormous in the very first year, and over the next three years predictions that were initially called alarmist proved to be underestimates. The same situation exists today as the major cities, most impressively New York City, face severe bed shortages and shortages of health care workers. While the resistance to funding at the federal, state, and local levels of government is hardly unique in the nation's history, it does require explanation, especially since for the first five years of the epidemic it seemed entirely possible that the disease would spread steadily into the heterosexual population, thus quite directly threatening majority groups.

The foundations do not appear to have a much better record than that of federal, state, and local governments. At least that is what can be gleaned from the carefully researched but cautiously phrased

14. State funding patterns for AIDS vary greatly. One study found that California's expenditures per cumulative AIDS case between 1983 and 1986 were 100 percent higher than the national average, while New York's reached only 45 percent of the national average. See Intergovernmental Health Policy Project, "State-Only Expenditures for AIDS: Major Trends, Fiscal Years 1983–1986," *Focus On*, no. 18 (October 1987). Another study noted that, as would be expected, states where party rivalry and the power of social conservatives are important spend less than average. Contrary to expectations, however, per capita income and rate of economic growth are also positively associated with below-average state expenditures per AIDS case. See David C. Colby and David G. Baker, "State Policy Responses."

publication by the Foundation Center, *AIDS Funding: A Guide to Giving by Foundations and Charitable Organizations*, edited by John Clinton.

Private foundation funding initiatives addressing HIV infection and AIDS are "a recent phenomenon in terms of scale."[15] That puts it delicately. The epidemic was designated as such in 1981; in 1983 five small grants were made by four foundations. By 1985 AIDS was being identified as the public health crisis of the century, but only sixty-eight foundations gave grants dealing with AIDS in 1986. As of August 1988, when the study under review was completed, there were 157. Half of the cumulative dollar value of some $51.6 million had come from the Robert Wood Johnson Foundation. Finally, only 3 percent of the foundations that annually award $100,000 or more in grants have funded AIDS.

Obviously, the need for funds is there. In the spring of 1988 the Robert Wood Johnson Foundation announced a new program and called for proposals. The proposals that were submitted asked for a total of $537 million (in a year when all foundation grants for AIDS totaled only $22.7 million—4 percent of the requests made in response to one mailing by one foundation, though the major one). With the federal government reportedly lavishing research funds on a small number of laboratories and researchers, it is fortunate that most of the current foundation funding is not directed to medical research; 53 percent is for medical care. Grants concerned with minority communities accounted for 20 percent of all grants until 1988, when the total amount of minority grants stayed the same but their proportion of all grants declined to 8 percent. Since it is in minority communities that the AIDS cases are expanding most rapidly, the proportion should have risen, perhaps to 40 percent or so. But fortunately foundation grants concerned with intravenous drug users and with women are both up, though they are equally small in size. The spread of AIDS among minorities, drug users, and their female partners is the most pressing problem and the most difficult to deal with. These would seem to be the most important groups for private foundations to attempt to reach, since the challenge is the great-

15. Foundation Center, *AIDS Funding*, p. ix.

est here and governments are hobbled by restrictions and red tape and have shown little enthusiasm for the task.

It is fruitless to ask what should have been the level of private and public foundation giving since the epidemic was announced in 1981. We have no precedent for this epidemic, and there is no national policy group for foundations giving the matter judicious thought and providing direction. Many foundations in the health area would have to change their basic policy to provide grants for a single disease.

We can say that the foundations were no later to enter the field than state governments were, and though the federal government spent a few million dollars in 1981–1983, from 1984 to 1988 the foundations increased their expenditures thirteen times faster than the federal and state governments. The big jump came from fiscal year (FY) 1986 to FY 1987, when spending went from $862,000 to $15,370,000; it rose to $22,692,000 in FY 1988. Should foundations be spending more than 2.8 percent of federal expenditures and 18 percent of state expenditures on the biggest health crisis of the century? Every study conducted, including the Presidential Commission report, the Institute of Medicine studies, and those of the major foundations, agrees that the federal and state governments should be spending vastly more. Perhaps the foundations should too.

INITIAL RESEARCH: EASY AND LATE

The AIDS research effort is almost universally applauded, and government publications routinely speak of the remarkable speed with which progress has already been made. Comparisons are made to diseases in the early part of the century, but they overlook the massive advantages in resources and knowledge we have now. As Shilts points out, the National Cancer Institute did not form a task force until April 1983, twenty-two months into the epidemic. Identifying the virus was not difficult. French researchers in the laboratory of Dr. Luc Montagnier at the Pasteur Institute isolated it in June 1983 after only a few months of research. But they could not grow it. Dr. Robert Gallo, whose research at the NCI began in the same year, isolated the same virus a year later, in

April 1984; he could grow it and claimed discovery. Since the French
sent crucial samples to Dr. Gallo, and the virus he identified was identical with these strains, an ugly priority dispute emerged, reaching up to
the heads of states of the respective nations. A "co-discovery" was
announced.[16] Dr. Jay Levy, of the University of California in San Francisco, was ready to announce that he too had discovered a virus at the
same time, after only eight months of research. Thus, the discoveries
came quickly once the work started. Shilts suggests that the problem
was not finding it but that it took so long for anyone to try.[17] (He also
documents more "normal" bureaucratic problems, such as fighting
between the research agencies, as does Panem in her book, and the
isolation of AIDS researchers by others in the University of California
medical schools and research hospitals. Once research money started
flowing, there were complaints that it was being syphoned from other
areas and that the largesse was somehow destabilizing. Gina Kolata, for
example, writing in *Science* magazine in 1983, spoke of a "surge of
research funds" from the federal government, which spent more on AIDS

16. Shilts, *And the Band Played On*, p. 593, notes that to say that Gallo and
Montagnier were co-discoverers is a "pleasant fiction." An extremely thorough,
dramatic, almost book-length account of the Gallo affair, with many more damaging materials regarding Gallo and the U.S. government than Shilts provides, appears
in the special report by John Crewdson, "The Great AIDS Quest," in the November 19, 1989, issue of the *Chicago Tribune*.

17. Typical of the upbeat view of research efforts is the General Accounting Office's
task force report, *Coping With AIDS in the Workplace*, which asserts that the "speed
with which progress has already been made is quite remarkable" (p. 23). The
Report of the Presidential Commission acknowledges that "Our national system of
research programming and funding is not equipped to reorganize rapidly in response
to an emergency" (p. 37) but adds, "The advances made to date in [AIDS] research
rest on a foundation of research excellence established many years ago at NIH and
accelerated in the 1970s by the 'War on Cancer'" (p. 38). On the discovery
process, see Shilts, *And the Band Played On*, pp. 271, 319, 450–452, and 529.

Panem, *AIDS Bureaucracy*, is almost breathless in her admiration for the speed
and success of the research effort. It is difficult to judge such matters, but the
detail that Shilts offers regarding the critical first three years suggests scant and
tardy effort. Since about 1984 both effort and progress have been increasingly
impressive, given the exceedingly "deceptive" character of the virus.

in one year than had been spent over eight years on Legionnaire's disease and toxic shock syndrome combined. But despite the "unprecedented spending spree," she notes that some scientists were organizing auctions and using other unorthodox devices to raise money for care or research. "AIDS, in fact, is so enormously intriguing to all sorts of scientists . . . that despite all the research money available, there is simply not enough to finance everyone who wants to get into the field." This was written at a time when the research budget of the Department of Health and Human Services (DHHS), which includes the National Institutes of Health (NIH) and the Centers for Disease Control, was only $14.5 million.[18]

EDUCATION STILL A FAILURE

In the realm of education programs the picture had not changed appreciably even by 1988. The first risk-reduction guideline by the Public Health Service (PHS) did not appear until T-21, March 1983, and there were just two sentences of guidance to gay men.[19] In the same year the PHS ruled that the hotline it set up could not counsel callers on sexual matters or even mention condoms. In late 1985 conservatives in the White House blocked the use of CDC money for education. In December 1987, a national TV network had to delete references to condoms on an education program because some of the financing came from the Department of Education. Meanwhile, the conservative government of Great Britain in late 1987 launched a "massive, sexually explicit education campaign."[20] As of 1987, the United States was the only major western nation without a national education program; some would say none really existed even in late 1989. In 1987, the General Accounting

18. Kolata, "Congress, NIH Open Coffers."
19. Shilts, *And the Band Played On*, p. 242. "Sexual contact should be avoided with persons known or suspected to have AIDS," the pronouncement stated. "Members of high-risk groups should be aware that multiple sexual partners increase the probability of developing AIDS." As Shilts notes, twenty months into the epidemic this is the sum total of the government's attempt to prevent the spread of the disease among gay men.
20. Turner, Miller, and Moses, eds., *AIDS*, p. 382.

Office reported to a Senate committee that "in each fiscal year since 1983 . . . congressional appropriations have consistently exceeded the administration's budget requests" and that "the administration's budget request of 155 million dollars [for fiscal 1988] does not provide sufficient funding for education of either the general public or targeted groups." The GAO also reported that "in fiscal year 1987 the Department of Defense spent $180 million for magazine and television advertising directed at new recruits and reservists."[21] In 1988 the U.S. Senate passed an amendment proposed by Senator Jesse Helms that limited the types of educational programs that could be funded with federal monies and that prohibited "the encouragement of homosexual activities."[22]

Conflicts among branches of the federal government have delayed education actions. The AIDS information brochure that should have been sent to every American household in 1987 stands as a monument to government paralysis and denial six years into an epidemic that had already taken the lives of 45,000 citizens. The long process of editing and review involved staff from the Public Health Service, the Office of the Assistant Secretary for Health and Human Services, the Domestic Policy Council, and the Office of Management and the Budget. Before the end of the year 45 million copies of the brochure, *What You Should Know about AIDS*, were actually printed. But the mailing did not start and was finally cancelled. It was not until June 1988 that the Public Health Service finally distributed a different brochure, *Understanding AIDS*. The most striking characteristic of these brochures is that, in the view of a study conducted for the National Research Council of the National Academy of Sciences, both confounded "moral advice with information" and failed to "communicate in a value-free manner with simple and explicit language that avoids moralizing." In the 1987 brochure, the word *gay* appeared only once, in a quotation from an AIDS outreach worker.[23]

California was the first state to initiate education programs, and its

21. General Accounting Office, *AIDS Prevention*, pp. 26 and 27.
22. Ronald Bayer, *Private Acts, Social Consequences*, p. 218.
23. Turner, Miller, and Moses, eds., *AIDS*, pp. 384–385.

story is instructive. It suggests that legislators are not as hostile as the argument that homophobia led to inaction might suggest. In 1983 sociologist Levi Kamel, who had been AIDS Education Director for the Los Angeles Gay and Lesbian Community Center, became the first California AIDS Education Services Director. California had already appropriated $500,000 for AIDS education—a princely sum given the response of the federal government and the nonresponse of New York State. At the first legislative hearing Kamel attended he interrupted his superior, who was saying what a good job had been done with the money and how the job was now finished, to make a twenty-minute speech about the diversity of the affected communities, the difficulty of changing pleasurable behaviors, and the need to educate and support caregivers as well as persons with AIDS. According to a senatorial staff member who was present, Kamel seemed to have "blown it" in his first appearance as a staff member. But suddenly the legislators were chiming in with comments such as "I haven't seen any billboards in my district, heard any Spanish radio spots in my district, learned of an outreach program in my district." They voted to double the appropriations for the next year.[24] A courageous outcry made the difference.

California was able to fund the education efforts of thirteen community-based groups in the next year, but outside of California there was very little education; the gay male community could not do much on its own. The few gay-run and gay-financed hotlines were overwhelmed with callers, according to our respondents in New York City. Coverage in the gay press was useful but consisted primarily of fierce debates about bathhouses, whether safe sex practices were necessary, and even whether there was an epidemic.[25] Perhaps the biggest educational breakthrough

24. Berg, "The AIDS Experience," p. 3.
25. Denial of the crisis might be expected from bathhouse owners, one of whom calculated that there had been 4 billion gay sexual encounters in 4.5 years but only 1,279 AIDS cases, concluding that the disease was not sexually transmitted (Shilts, p. 307). But scientists familiar with the patterns of epidemics should have known better, but even a sociologist, one year into the epidemic, could write that "278 cases out of a possible 11 million [gay men in America] hardly constitutes an epidemic" (Shilts, p. 167).

came in July 1985, when movie star Rock Hudson went public with his AIDS diagnosis (originally made fourteen months earlier). One suspects that the country needed someone with an otherwise splendid, masculine, and moral image to be affected before the disease could no longer be so easily dismissed as retribution for stigmatized behavior. The Hudson announcement was made shortly after he had videotaped an appearance for Doris Day's program on the Christian Broadcasting System. His credentials were impeccable.

EDUCATION TO CHANGE RISKY BEHAVIOR

We believe that a vigorous education campaign in the first year of the epidemic could have saved several thousand lives. Changing gay men's sexual behavior was a priority for some medical people from the start, but individual and organizational resistance was strong among gays. Despite early evidence that the disease was being spread by a few highly active homosexual men, largely through gay clubs and the bathhouses of San Francisco and New York, the gay community (and the owners of the profitable bathhouses) resisted any restraints on its behavior. In his detailed account of the bathhouse polemic, Ronald Bayer, a professor at Columbia University's School of Public Health, documents the inaction of the gay press and such influential groups as the Gay Men's Health Crisis (GMHC), which bluntly refused even to talk about regulating or conducting education campaigns at the bathhouses.[26] There were, however, many gay physicians and groups, like the National Gay Task Force, pressing for some sort of regulation.[27] Public health officials were also cautious to an extreme, perhaps because of gay political pressure or the controversial nature of the establishments and of such drastic action. In any case, the bathhouses remained open during the first three years of the epidemic.

Closing the houses was not discussed seriously until May 1982, eleven months into the crisis. As late as May 1983, when the country had

26. Bayer, *Private Acts, Social Consequences*, pp. 30 and 54.
27. Bayer, pp. 54–55.

1,450 reported cases, 45 percent of them in New York City, an official of that city rejected suggestions for education, saying that gay men were providing it themselves, and turned aside concerns about the bathhouses with the libertarian argument that the "city should not tell people how to have sex." By February 1985 the city's AIDS cases surpassed 3,000, yet the New York City Health Commissioner, Dr. David Sencer, maintained that education was adequate and dismissed the idea that there was a crisis in New York City. Governor Mario Cuomo of New York, a liberal Democrat, assured gay leaders that the bathhouses would not be closed and, for the second year in a row, opposed allocating any funds to fight AIDS.[28] Owners resisted any suggestion that bathhouses should be the location for education regarding AIDS and had to be ordered to put up warning posters. (The resistance to posters was based not only on a commercial argument but also on a civil liberties argument; a similar resistance by the National Organization of Women to posters in bars warning women about the effects of alcohol on the fetus was based on the right to privacy.) San Francisco bathhouses were ordered to put up warning posters in June 1983, but a survey in March 1984 indicated only feeble compliance. Closings started in September 1984 (T-39) in San Francisco, and bathhouses were closed in many cities in the rest of the nation by mid-1985, though they remained open in Los Angeles, at least.

Closing the houses was clearly not easy. The Director of Public Health in San Francisco during this period was Dr. Mervyn Silverman, who later was co-founder of the American Foundation for AIDS Research (AmFAR). Initially he was against closings but favored regulation.[29] He later changed his mind and in October 1984 ordered the closing of the gay bathhouses and clubs, but the civil liberties issues were serious. A few weeks after the closings a superior court ordered that they be reopened on the ground that public health and civil liberties concerns should be balanced,[30] although one gay physician, Marcus Conant, testified that

28. Shilts, pp. 310, 455, 533; Bayer, pp. 32, 38, 59–61.
29. Bayer, pp. 50–53.
30. Bayer, pp. 50–53. A detailed account of the constitutional aspects of AIDS may be found in Rabin, "The AIDS Epidemic and Gay Bathhouses."

some gay men infected at bathhouses would return to them and "not feel guilty about giving it back."[31] But Silverman, a vigorous advocate for more education and more care, offered a striking observation a year later in an interview with Sandra Panem. Silverman said that Dianne Feinstein, then mayor of San Francisco and very supportive of the gay population, had remarked, "'If this had been a heterosexual disease, I would have closed the bathhouses immediately.' And she's right, because it wouldn't have been a bathhouse; it would have been a whorehouse," and that would be easier to close. Presumably Silverman meant that straight "johns" were not as well organized as gay men.[32]

One argument against closing bathhouses was that frequent anonymous anal sex would "go underground." As Shilts notes with bitter irony, however, sodomy in public parks and neighborhood bushes by "unrestrained sex fiends," predicted even by New York State Commissioner of Health David Axelrod, who initially opposed the closings, did not occur.[33] The opportunity to use the houses as places to inform highly active homosexual men of the risk—something most bathhouse owners strongly resisted because it would undoubtedly diminish the attraction of the institutions and reduce their profits—not only was never realized, but was probably unlikely from the start. At least one bathhouse in New York City handed out condoms and displayed posters, according to a GMHC official, but there is no evidence that a serious effort was made. It was not until October 1985 that Axelrod and Cuomo, side by side, announced the closing of the bathhouses. In New York City, Mayor Koch and Commissioner Sencer decided to postpone implementation of the new state directive and were moved to act only under direct pressure from Albany.[34]

The problem of highly efficient transmission of the virus through central locations such as bathhouses persists and probably always will. A survey in 1986 of 807 men leaving seven bathhouses in Los Angeles

31. Bayer, pp. 47–48.
32. Panem, *AIDS Bureaucracy*, pp. 19–20.
33. Shilts, pp. 453–454.
34. Bayer, pp. 62–64.

found that while all but 2 percent reported familiarity with the AIDS information that was distributed in the bathhouses, 10 percent continued to practice anal intercourse without a condom. These were likely to be the poorer, younger, less-educated members of the sample (though the patrons as a whole were prosperous), and they were more likely to have had five or more partners in the previous month.[35] From 2,000 to 4,000 males visited bathhouses in the Los Angeles area each week. Bathhouses remained closed, technically, in New York City, but some gay cinemas and clubs apparently provided opportunities for risky sex at the close of the 1980s (and may still). One gay cinema, recently closed after repeated warnings, had, among other things, provisions for the "glory holes" that were featured in the San Francisco Castro district in the 1970s.[36] These are plywood partitions with holes cut into them, to permit thoroughly anonymous anal sex on a production-line basis. It is hard to conceive of a more efficient transmission device; it is even harder to see how it could operate in 1988, given all the publicity about AIDS. Obviously more than education is required to convince *everyone* to give up risky behavior. But an epidemic cannot be sustained if there are only a *few* sources of transmission.

The dynamics of epidemics are somewhat counterintuitive. High success rates with prevention efforts are not necessary to stop the epidemic, though they are needed to eliminate the risk for specific individuals. For an epidemic to be sustained it is necessary that every infected person has

35. Richwald et al., "Sexual Activities in Bathhouses."
36. McFadden, "Health Department Closes Down Gay Cinema." The owners of the establishment acknowledged to city officials that they were aware of the risky sexual practices and would assign personnel to "discourage sexual activity among the patrons." But they left in place, and in use, seven cubicles and partitions with small holes to accommodate anonymous contacts. Thomas B. Stoddard, executive director of Lambda Legal Defense and Education Fund, objected to the closing of the cinema: "We generally oppose all acts of this kind by the government. Consensual sexual activity by adults out of public view should always be beyond the eye and the arm of the government." Two other gay cinemas were closed a few months later. The action was opposed by gay rights advocates and the New York Civil Liberties Union. See Wait, "New York Shuts 2 Gay Theatres."
On the Castro scene, see Fitzgerald, *Cities on a Hill*, pp. 25–119.

to infect, on average, one other. Because there is a good chance that a fair proportion of the sexual contacts will occur between already infected individuals, however, an infected person contacting a variety of people in a well-defined social group will not be sustaining the epidemic if all are infected. To sustain the epidemic, therefore, those outside the group have to infect more than one person, enough to make up for those who are either not infecting anyone or contacting only those already infected. No one gets well, of course; the disease still spreads; but if it does not spread in epidemic terms it will eventually die out as the number of carriers declines.[37]

⌈In addition to closing down transmission sites, an education campaign directed to the private physicians who serve the gay male population and to the sexually transmitted disease (STD) clinics could have prevented thousands of subsequent infections. Mass media education campaigns, while necessary, are the least effective; the most needed campaigns are those that target the most concentrated sources of infection. The presumably small proportion of the gay male population that engages in very frequent casual sex is also the population with the highest rate of sexually transmitted diseases, such as hepatitis B, syphilis, gonorrhea, and genital warts. There are successful treatments for these diseases, so these individuals visit their doctors fairly regularly. A concerted, well-funded campaign to persuade the doctors to convince their patients that they were in danger of contracting a debilitating and presumably fatal disease, and of spreading it to their partners, could have made a large difference. Even if only one-third of the highly active population took precautions or limited their participation in risky forms of sexual behavior, the spread would have been greatly reduced.

But no significant effort was made to launch an educational campaign

37. The dynamics of the AIDS epidemic was first explored in May and Anderson, "Transmission Dynamics." Edward H. Kaplan and his co-authors have explored the policy implications of intervention strategies with reference to the important but neglected matter of sexual mixing and the high utility of even quite imperfect education programs. See Kaplan, "Can Bad Models Suggest Good Policies?"; and Kaplan and Abramson, "So What If the Program Ain't Perfect?" The classic (and fascinating) historical discussion of epidemics is McNeill, *Plagues and Peoples*.

that would reach doctors who treat gay men. Nor was any substantial effort made to flood the STD clinics with counselors or at least literature on the new risk. In those early days—say, from 1982 to 1984, when the epidemic first became apparent—most of the at-risk population was visible, accessible, and geographically concentrated in small sections of New York City and San Francisco. As AIDS spread at a slower rate into the gay population that engaged in progressively less frequent and casual sex, the difficulties of effective education increased. It was simply not inevitable that about half of all gay men in San Francisco and New York City would become HIV-positive, as estimates still suggest. Reaching the other major group, the IVDUs, would have been much more difficult, but even here it was not inevitable that from 60 to 90 percent of New York City's IVDUs would be infected (estimates vary widely). The rate in cities that are not on the East Coast is believed to be only about 5 percent.[38]

The education failure rests upon the gay community, the medical community, and above all upon public officials. The gay community was initially reluctant to recognize the problems with disseminating sources and risky behavior, but within a couple of years it was conducting educational efforts, and for several years these efforts were the only meaningful ones. The doctors in San Francisco and New York City who included gay men among their patients, and especially those that specialized in sexually transmitted diseases in males, appear to have made no organized effort to educate even their clients, let alone the population from which their clients were drawn. But the most serious failure is that of public health officials and public officials in general. For a top health official in New York City to declare proudly that he was not about to tell gay men how to have sex, when this was exactly what was needed, was to commit thousands to death. Nor can these criticisms be dismissed as hindsight. As Shilts's history of the early days repeatedly demonstrates, responsible people, including public officials, spoke out for the need for aggressive education. Nor would an education campaign have to have been 90 percent or even 50 percent effective to make a decisive difference.

Doctors' offices should have been flooded with literature about the

38. Mahar, "Pitiless Scourge," p. 16.

risk. A special team should have been formed in at least the two major cities to contact these doctors, and informational packets should have been provided for them to send privately to their patients. The STD clinics should have had the same sort of literature and increases in staff as well. Special counselors should have been hired to alert gay men and spouses and lovers of IVDUs (among whom hepatitis B is widespread). The organized gay community, instead of being ignored as they clamored for help, should have been enlisted to arrange special parties, meetings, and mailings. There was great controversy over the degree of danger, the amount of denial, and the behavioral sources of risk, but government tried to avoid taking a stand. AIDS came at a time when state and municipal budgets were beginning to expand again;[39] pleading poverty, as Governor Cuomo did, for example, was mere expediency.

The education of gay men was bound to be difficult, and it is far from accomplished. There are areas of New York City today where men cruise in cars to pick up young men who sell themselves, and presumably condoms are not used. The success of the educational efforts even from a presumably trusted source, the gay community itself, is difficult to judge. Though the examples are not strictly comparable, the judgment should be in terms of efforts to persuade teenagers to use condoms (dismal success) and the campaigns against smoking, excessive drinking, excessive eating, gambling, and drug abuse — in short, to change lifestyles and sources of instant gratification. Behavioral changes in these areas, even under the threat of death in a few years, will not come easily. Education must be massive and explicit.

The record for changing drug-taking or sexual behavior for IVDUs, gay or heterosexual, appears to be dismal. Compounding this difficulty is the fact that the disease is transmitted more efficiently through needle sharing than through sexual activity.[40] An even more serious problem was the refusal of New York City's health officials even to try. A 1985

39. Between 1982 and 1986 state and city government budgets grew at approximately the same rate as the Gross National Product, both in the nation as a whole and in New York. Renshaw, Trott, and Friedenberg, "Gross State Product by Industry, 1963–1986."
40. Kaplan, "Needles That Kill."

mayoral report from Health Commissioner Sencer said that drug users are "unlikely to change their risk behavior" and that "prevention of transmission in this population is unlikely." This was the same year in which Deputy Mayor Victor Botnick was quoted as saying "New York City has no epidemic, no AIDS crisis," and Patricia Maher, a member of the city's AIDS staff, quit in protest over the refusal to put warnings in subways. She was told that anybody who needs to know about AIDS already knows about it.[41]

The record for gay men is mixed, but on balance, the majority (but perhaps only a modest majority) appear to have changed their sexual behavior. For example, the rate of rectal gonorrhea fell quickly as gay men began using condoms—on the other hand, condom sales increased only 94 percent in four years and now has leveled off. Since condoms should be used by both gay men and heterosexuals, we might have wished for much more growth.[42] A survey of five hundred gay men in October 1984, forty months into the epidemic and before the bathhouses were closed, found that two-thirds had changed their sexual habits enough to remove any risk of contracting the infection.[43] In San Francisco, the proportion of gay men practicing insertive anal intercourse decreased from 40 percent in 1985 to 14 percent in 1987, and the average number of sexual partners per year had declined by 20 percent in one sample survey. A 1986 study among gay men in New York City found that the average number of sexual partners per year decreased from thirty-six prior to the onset of the epidemic to eight when it became clear that multiple partners increased the chances of infection.[44] Fifty-nine percent of IVDUs interviewed in a New York methadone clinic as early as 1984 reported some sort of behavior change to avoid infection, and a survey in 1985 found identical results.[45] The figures are only suggestive and prob-

41. Lambert, "Koch's Record on AIDS."
42. Mahar, "Pitiless Scourge," p. 16.
43. Shilts, p. 492.
44. Marshall H. Becker and Jill G. Joseph have summarized recent research findings concerning behavioral adaptations for coping with the risks of getting AIDS in "AIDS and Behavioral Change."
45. Becker and Joseph, p. 403.

ably exaggerate the amount of change. For one thing, the samples of gay men and IVDUs are from those most accessible to education and to change, either because they are in or seeking treatment or because they are willing to be interviewed in fairly public settings, such as outside bathhouses. We have no data on young men just beginning to engage in gay sex, on practicing homosexuals in general, or on bisexuals who are married or still "in the closet" in areas outside the major cities such as San Francisco, New York, Miami, and Los Angeles. The belief that sexual freedom is essential to a gay life-style has been found to be related to higher numbers of sexual partners and hence to increased risk of infection.[46]

Mathilde Krim, co-founder of the American Foundation for AIDS Research, told the following story to Maggie Mahar:

> Where homosexuality is less accepted than it is in New York or San Francisco, the disease could spread more insidiously: A community inclined to deny homosexuality is also denying the danger of AIDS. Recently, I gave a talk at the University of Utah and I noticed no official representatives of the local gay community in the audience. Usually, they are there when I talk. But in the back of the audience, I did notice three young men sitting together in a group, and I went up to them and asked who they were. They replied, "We're the gay community." "Just three of you?" I asked. "The rest are married," they said. That morning the Salt Lake City newspaper reported the case of a young mother diagnosed with AIDS. The article said she had no idea how she could have contracted the disease.[47]

As long as homosexual orientation is penalized, some young homosexual men are likely to be isolated from knowledge of STDs, including AIDS; and since monogamous homosexual relations are not exempt from social stigma, more easily concealed promiscuous relations in effect are encouraged. It is clear that the education of young homosexual men,

46. Becker and Joseph, p. 395.
47. Mahar, p. 16.

especially those who were still children in the 1980s, when AIDS had such dramatic impact on the gay community, will not be easy.[48] The Institute for the Protection of Lesbian and Gay Youth in New York City recently found that attendance at its weekly discussion group dropped from fifty to two when it was announced that the subject would be AIDS. The topics generally involved "relationships," sexuality, dating, and even drugs. AIDS could be dealt with only if it was integrated into these "more comfortable" topics, we were told, which is what the institute then did.

We are only beginning to get information about the new wave of crack addiction, which presents a most formidable problem of educating female addicts who exchange sex for drugs. A recent study showed that 35 to 40 percent of those entering crack houses had previous experience with intravenous drug use. Crack houses foster marathon binges of cocaine use and a variety of sexual activities, sometimes with dozens of partners for two days or more. There is also an alarming rise in syphilis in the populations most vulnerable to crack addiction: in New York City, while it has dropped among white males in the past five years, it has increased by 150 percent among blacks, 73 percent among Hispanics, and more than doubled among women.[49] The combination of crack binges, prolonged bouts of sex, HIV-positive IVDUs, and syphilis, it is feared, will lead to the spread of AIDS in a heterosexual population that is all but invulnerable to even the most forceful education programs (though no study has yet documented that syphilis sores are effective transmission routes). But a concerted effort starting in 1981 or 1982 to bring more IVDUs into methadone treatment centers and educate them about the transmission of AIDS through shared needles and unprotected sex would have reduced the size of the present crisis and the number of its carriers. What might appear to be a virtually hopeless education task now, with the spread of AIDS into the minority community through complex inter-

48. Scientists are divided as to whether sexual orientation is genetic or acquired, but homosexuality is no longer associated with "mental illness" or "moral failure." See Risman and Schwartz, "Sociological Research on Male and Female Homosexuality."

49. Kerr, "Syphilis Surge and Crack Use Raising Fears."

actions (infected IVDUs, crack houses, syphilis, homelessness), was certainly more tractable in the early years.

AIDS is the only epidemic for which the means of prevention are available in the local supermarket, are cheap, and are easy to use. The resistance to using condoms and bleach or alcohol is, in one sense, extraordinary. Forgoing sex or breaking a drug habit (or forgoing the occasional injection) is admittedly harder, but neither is even necessary to avoid AIDS. An education campaign that said your life could depend upon using a condom when practicing anal sex, and flushing your syringe out with bleach or alcohol and rinsing with water before shooting up, would have been very cheap and very successful in saving lives. But such campaigns were not tried in the United States. The risk of encouraging nonmarital sex or IVDU by publicizing supermarket remedies was seen by powerful groups as worse than the risk of an epidemic of deaths.

Responsible people called for massive education; it could have had a substantial effect; it is still needed. European countries, though experiencing the epidemic later and so far in much smaller numbers, did a far better job. It is a job for organizations. They failed in a massive way, and later we shall discuss why.

THE BLOOD INDUSTRY

Our final example of the failure of organizations concerns the blood industry, both the for-profit and the nonprofit organizations and their trade groups. The critical dates are given in Table 2-1. Blood was suspected to be the transmission agent from the beginning, and in July 1982, T-13, the CDC warned the blood industry of the problem and asked the blood banks not to accept blood from high-risk groups—gay men and IVDUs. In August 1982, T-14, it also recommended to the Public Health Service that all blood be tested for evidence of hepatitis B with a core antibody test (rather than the one routinely used), since there was a very high correlation between signs of the new disease and evidence of hepatitis B (which is a blood-borne virus very common among both gay men and IVDUs). And in December 1982 the first fully documented transfusion case, the "smoking gun," was available. It was believed that homosexual men contributed disproportionately to the blood supply; thus the supply could be quickly contaminated, as it indeed was. Given the lack of knowledge on the nature of the virus, which was not determined until April 1984, a blood test to screen infected donations was still unattainable. Screening high-risk donors was the only, imperfect solution available. In March 1983, the PHS proposed that donors from high-risk groups voluntarily refrain from donating blood and plasma in the future.[50]

Nevertheless, the gay male community strongly opposed screening for high-risk groups on civil rights grounds, and the blood industry denied the danger. In January 1983, T-19, seven months after the first warning and one month after the first fully documented case, the president of the New York Blood Center said there was no evidence that the virus was transmitted through blood or blood products. A year later the Red Cross repeated that statement despite an article by CDC researchers published in the *New England Journal of Medicine* documenting transfusion-associated cases of AIDS. In March 1984, T-33, the president of the New York Blood Center still denied transmission by blood and, more important, still refused to test for hepatitis B as the CDC had recommended eighteen months previously. In December 1984 there were ninety documented cases of AIDS caused by blood transfusions and forty-nine cases of AIDS infection due to contamination of the blood-clotting factor used by hemophiliacs. In March 1985, the first blood test for antibodies to HIV was available and put to use, but even this did not end the denial and delay.

Two further problems remained: whether donors who test positive should be notified (their donated blood would not be used for transfusions in any event), and whether blood banks should investigate previous donations by donors now found to be infected. Both concerns touched on the possibility that people infected by a blood transfusion, before the availability of the screening test, might unwittingly spread the virus. Because the first test available, the enzyme-linked immunosorbent assay

50. The safety thus provided was later found to be fairly limited. One study reported that 20 percent of HIV-positive gay male donors had not acknowledged their homosexual orientation when asked by blood-screening personnel. See Bayer, *op. cit.*, p. 98.

Table 2-1. *A chronology of events related to the management of the blood supply*

T	Month	Year	
00	JUN	81	First Centers for Disease Control (CDC) report on the disease
06	DEC	81	Blood suspected; three infants with IVDU parents
13	JUL	82	Three hemophilia cases; first CDC warning to blood industry
14	AUG	82	CDC asks blood banks not to accept high-risk donors; CDC recommends hepatitis B blood testing to Public Health Service (PHS)
18	DEC	82	First fully documented transfusion case by CDC
19	JAN	83	President of New York Blood Center denies evidence of transmission
21	MAR	83	PHS guidelines: persons from high-risk groups asked to refrain voluntarily from donating blood and plasma, but CDC's recommended hepatitis B blood screening is still not required
31	JAN	84	American Red Cross still minimizes transmission danger; *New England Journal of Medicine* article written by CDC scientists documents transfusion-associated cases of AIDS
33	MAR	84	New York Blood Center president still denies transmission; center still does not do the kind of testing CDC recommends
34	APR	84	Retrovirus HTLV-III identified as responsible for AIDS; test to protect blood supply now foreseeable
42	DEC	84	90 cases of transfusion AIDS; 49 Factor VIII hemophiliac cases of AIDS infection (clotting factor)
45	MAR	85	First blood test for AIDS (ELISA); blood banks begin screening but do not notify positive donors unless the more accurate and more expensive Western blot test is conducted on the ELISA-positive blood samples
48	JUN	85	Citing the possibility of making errors, the American Association of Blood Banks, American Red Cross, and Council of Community Blood Centers agree not

Table 2-1. continued

T	Month	Year	
			to initiate a "lookback" program to identify blood recipients and notify them that their past donor(s) have now been found to be infected with HIV; no statute or regulation requires lookbacks
49	JUL	85	Notification of test results to donors begins
50	AUG	85	National Institutes of Health says blood screening has been successful
53	NOV	85	Thousands of people begin storing their own blood for future therapeutic transfusions
58	APR	86	Blood agencies decide to reverse their June 1985 decision and proceed with the "lookback" program
60	JUN	86	First CDC report of a patient infected with AIDS from a blood transfusion that had been tested; blood test known to be sensitive only 95 percent of the time
61	JUL	86	Greater New York Blood Program tries to identify 700 people who since 1977 received transfusions of blood that might be infected
74	AUG	87	New York Blood Center claims it was the first to be on top of issue and denies knowledge of blood contamination by AIDS was available before spring of 1983
83	MAY	88	Nearly 7,500 U.S. hemophiliacs believed to be infected with HIV
90	DEC	88	Irwin Memorial Blood Bank in San Francisco is the first in U.S. to be successfully sued for negligence in providing infected blood for a transfusion in 1983
94	APR	89	900 hemophiliac and 2,300 blood-transfusion AIDS cases reported already to CDC; hundreds of lawsuits filed against blood banks

(ELISA), was especially designed to have an extremely high proportion of false positives (sometimes as high as 40 percent), so as to protect the blood supply effectively, blood bankers refused to notify ELISA-positive donors of their condition. (Of course, they did not use the donated blood for transfusions.) There were other tests available, like the Western blot technique, a confirmatory test far more accurate and reliable than ELISA but also much more expensive. Thus, the blood industry preferred to risk the unwitting transmission of the virus by some unknown proportion of the donors the ELISA test had found to be seropositive by never notifying them of their possible condition. (The Red Cross later designed a cost-effective strategy which consisted in administering the Western blot test to the blood samples that had tested positive for ELISA.) It was not until July 1985, T-49, or three months after the first test was available, that the result of the ELISA test was given to the donating person. This happened only when blood bankers became more familiar with and confident of the application of the test.[51]

The second remaining problem involved more serious charges against the for-profit and nonprofit blood industry—withholding (or not seeking out) information. Representatives of the American Association of Blood Banks, the American Red Cross, and the Council of Community Blood Centers issued a joint statement in June 1985, T-48, in which they agreed not to track back the donation histories of donors now found to be infected with the virus. This program would have helped to identify past blood recipients who might have been infected and could have been passing on the virus ever since. The blood bankers argued that a "lookback" program would involve many errors and that, as a result, "the injury to prior recipients which may be caused by such [erroneous] notification is disproportionate to the benefits, which are tenuous and ill-defined." As Bayer notes, had the blood banks conducted the program from the moment the test was available, the associated costs "would have posed yet another administrative burden that blood bankers were not anxious to assume." Finally, almost a year later, in April of 1986, T-58, the blood agencies reversed their earlier decision and began the lookback program. After just three months of search, the Greater New

51. Bayer, *Private Acts, Social Consequences*, p. 96.

York Blood Program announced that it was trying to identify seven hundred people who received transfusions since 1977 and were thought to have been tainted with the virus. The lookback program thus proved to be a necessary step to protect the population at large.[52]

But denial of the possibility of a tainted blood supply has not completely ended; the historian of the epidemic will not have an easy time. Stanford University Hospital recognized the need for intervention and started an elaborate testing program in May 1983. But in March 1984, as noted above, the New York Blood Center was still denying that transmission by blood was possible. When we interviewed an official of the center in 1987 he claimed that the center was the first to be on top of the transfusion issue and that it was not until the spring of 1983 that there was knowledge of blood contamination by HIV-seropositive donors — both false statements.[53]

Screening high-risk donors was a controversial matter because gay men and addicts would be asked to disclose their risky or illegal behavior, and this information could be used (and surely was used in some cases) as grounds to fire them from their jobs or otherwise discriminate against them. (Homosexual acts are considered criminal offenses in about half the states.) An employee of an organization who was under any sort of suspicion of being gay or an addict would be confirming the suspicion and risking discharge if he refused to give blood for fear of infecting others. The matter eventually was easily solved by an instruction to add a checkmark to the form indicating that the blood was to be used for research purposes only. Though there was still some chance that the

52. Bayer, pp. 72–89, 98. On management of the blood supply, see Shilts, especially pp. 115–116, 160–163, 168–171, 220–226, 299–301, 307–309, 409–411, and 432–435. Panem, *AIDS Bureaucracy*, pp. 21–25, follows her practice of taking at face value the statements of the establishment, e.g., the representative of the American Association of Blood Banks.

53. Denial in the blood issue was the major factor behind the spread of AIDS into Japan, a country with negligible gay and IVDU populations. "A disbelief that AIDS could trouble Japan" lies behind the critical delay of over a year in taking adequate action to safeguard the blood supply. Imported American blood has recently been held responsible for a sizable number of hemophiliac AIDS cases. Said one infected person, "I cannot forgive that they continued selling to Japanese what had been forbidden to sell to Americans." Hiatt, "Tainted U.S. Blood Blamed."

employer, insurance company, or relatives might find out, this practice seems to have worked well.[54]

It is hard to account for the resistance and delay of the blood industry to test for hepatitis B as an indicator of AIDS-contaminated blood, its avoidance of the more expensive but also more reliable tests, and its decision at first not to check whether a seropositive donor had donated blood in the past. The cost of such testing would not have been great and would have been recovered by a rise in the price of blood. Blood has a highly inelastic demand, so the rise in cost would not affect profits. Even the more elaborate testing for the ratio of helper to suppressor lymphocytes, developed at Stanford University Hospital and required there in May 1983, increased the price of each blood unit by only six dollars, or about 10 percent.[55] Shilts reports an estimate that at least 12,000 people became HIV-positive during the period in which the blood could have been tested but wasn't.[56] We suspect it was the association of life-giving blood with dreaded AIDS that produced such vigorous denial and resistance.

54. Some problems remain, however. The HTLV-III / LAV antibody test currently used produces both false negative and false positive results. The former are said to be extremely rare (one in every 250,000), but the test is not reliable until four to six months after exposure to the HIV. Thus false negatives may not be as rare as the figure suggests. False positives are not rare in any case. Some studies have even found that 5 percent of positives are false. Roughly one-third of Americans currently believe that the blood supply is not safe (Johanna Pindyck, "AIDS and the Blood Service System"). New studies suggest that available tests may not detect some HIV carriers for years (see Kolata, "AIDS Test").

55. Shilts, p. 308.

56. Shilts, p. 599. The difference between Shilts's extensive account of the blood issue and the report by Johanna Pindyck, senior vice president of the New York Blood Center and director of the Greater New York Blood Program, is substantial. For example, according to Pindyck, blood banks have screened for hepatitis B since the 1970s; but this is an antibody test. The one that the CDC wanted and the blood industry refused to do was a core hepatitis test that detected the virus itself. As late as March 1984 Dr. Aaron Kellner of the New York Blood Center said the center refused to do core hepatitis testing, not because of cost but because it was not convinced that AIDS is transmitted by blood transfusion (Shilts, p. 433; Pindyck, "AIDS and the Blood Service System").

3   BUREAUCRATIC, ECONOMIC, AND

IDEOLOGICAL EXPLANATIONS

We have asserted that the federal government failed to fund education, research, and care; that the gay male community failed to warn and educate and change behavior quickly; that state and local governments failed to respond quickly; and that the blood industry failed to insure the safety of their product. How might this record be accounted for? The initial failure of the gay community could be readily explained in terms of their fear and panic, defensiveness in the face of hostility and stigma, and political marginality. In any case, the gay community soon responded with warnings, education, care, and behavioral changes. But the failure of government agencies and of the health sector in general is more surprising. Their poor record could be a matter of normal organizational failure—that is, of bureaucracy, the first of three explanations considered in this chapter. A second is economics. The inadequate response of the political and health sectors might be attributed to the heavy costs to be borne by the blood industry, bathhouse owners, and city governments, and more generally as an unacceptable challenge to the fiscal policies and philosophy of the Reagan administration, which was unwilling to institute or to spend money for a new federal health program.

There is a third possible explanation: the influence of a vigorous "moral majority" lobby that opposed action by the administration with which it was allied, though it could not affect the gay male groups or the blood industry so directly. All these explanations are important and will now be explored. Later we will argue that what made them more effective than usual was the unique nature of the disease itself. The specific characteristics of AIDS gave more force to these three explanations and added "synergy," the unexpected interaction of multiple failures, and increased the vulnerability of organizations to failure.

THE NORMAL FAILURE OF ORGANIZATIONS

Organizations are always failing to some degree, for they are imperfect and refractory tools.[1] The American health sector is particularly prone to failure. The United States spends more money per capita on health care and gets less results in aggregate good health statistics than any other industrialized nation. The public health system is highly fragmented, and the division of funding and services into a public and a private sphere is recognized as counterproductive by virtually all experts. In 1988 the Institute of Medicine issued a report, *The Future of Public Health*, painting a bleak portrait of a system in disarray, a system characterized by fragmented services, poor national leadership, and a complacent public. The slow response to the AIDS crisis is a symptom of a sickly health sector. "Who knows what crisis will be next?" asked the chairman of the committee that produced this report.[2]

AIDS fell upon a "system" that could tolerate only small-scale disturbances, such as Legionnaires disease or toxic shock syndrome, and that bungled its response to the epidemic that never was, swine flu.[3] Moreover, AIDS appeared after a time of high inflation and during a period of large federal cutbacks in poverty programs, housing, health

---

1. For a "refractory tool" view of organizations and their proneness to failure, see Perrow, *Complex Organizations*; and Perrow, *Normal Accidents*.
2. On the performance of national health care sectors, see Schieber, *Financing and Delivering Health Care*. For an analysis of the health care sector in New York City, see Paine, ed., *Health Care in Big Cities*; and Piore, Lieberman, and Linnane, "Public Expenditures and Private Control?" See also Institute of Medicine, *The Future of Public Health*.
3. For a particularly good account of the recent swine flue scare and the government's fumbling response, see Dutton, *Worse Than the Disease*.

care, and social services. Federal attempts to stem Medicare costs resulted in the "DRG" (diagnosis-related groups) program, which cut payments to hospitals. With reduced revenues, the hospitals had less slack to draw on when a surge of both mental patients and AIDS patients arrived in the mid-1980s. The fragile and inefficient health care system of the nation was thus subjected to multiple assaults. Even without the stigma and other unusual aspects of AIDS there would probably have been a number of sizable organizational failures. Even if the blood industry or organized gay men's groups or city politicians had responded quickly and effectively, the failing health sector, and especially the hospitals responsible for acute care, might have insured a disastrous overall response to the epidemic.

In the United States, in contrast to other industrialized nations, the hospitals are the focal point of the health care system. They are so important because we do so little in the way of preventive care; because physicians prefer to work out of hospitals rather than from their offices when possible; because we are more likely than other nations to use hospitals for routine procedures; and because the poor do not have physicians and so use the emergency facilities of hospitals. But the hospitals have been hit bad by the AIDS epidemic.

First, it has been estimated that private and public teaching hospitals, where many of the AIDS patients go, are reimbursed for just 76 percent of the hospitalization costs of an AIDS patient who has some private or government insurance. Two authorities, Lawrence Shulman and Joanne Mantell, argue that "hospitals have borne this burden and are losing significant amounts of money because of unreimbursed costs."[4] They call for alternative locations for acute "PWAs" (persons with AIDS) and alternative means of financing that spread the burden. Hospitals, they argue, cannot be blamed for the inadequate response to the AIDS crisis because their financial problems prevent an adequate response. Further-

4. Shulman and Mantell, in "The AIDS Crisis," emphasize the need to find and implement alternatives to hospitalization of PWAs for acute care and to involve communities and government at all levels in order to share the soaring hospital costs for AIDS patients.

more, they note, AIDS has affected hospitals in other negative ways. Hospitals with a specialized AIDS unit may experience "mass defection of nonAIDS patients who go elsewhere for medical care."[5] In addition, inner-city areas have experienced cutbacks in hospital beds because of an "overbedding crisis" that occurred as the suburbs built their own community and for-profit hospitals. The bed crisis in New York City is severe.

Thus, it might be argued that even a major epidemic of the nonpoor, nonstigmatized mainstream—for example, one that stemmed from widespread groundwater pollution and particularly affected the affluent suburbs—would have produced a number of organizational failures in the health care sector. We would have had instant hospital overcrowding, aggravating an existing shortage of nurses and prompting a financing crisis; an underfunded research establishment would have fumbled the research efforts; an image-conscious blood industry would have resisted testing the blood supply; and there would certainly be a shortage of nursing homes and hospices.

Timing is also crucial. The American health care sector has been undergoing major changes in recent decades, and AIDS joined and contributed to an ongoing crisis. Daniel Fox, a medical historian, discusses a number of important changes in recent decades that prevent effective management of an epidemic the size of AIDS. He notes the following relevant issues: changes in the causes of sickness and death that have required changes in facilities (for example, the increase in chronic diseases and the decline in infectious diseases); ambivalence about the recent progress of medical research and expensive life-extending procedures; a growing belief that people should take more responsibility for their own health (the "life-style" issue); a concern with uncontrollable rising costs; a policy that links health insurance "to employment rather than to membership in society"; and an increase in the power of for-profit health institutions, in the role of corporations in health benefits, and in the role of states as the federal government withdrew, all three contributing to a

5. Shulman and Mantell, "The AIDS Crisis"; for another expression of concern over this issue, see Fineberg, "The Social Dimensions of AIDS."

crisis of authority. As a consequence, Fox believes, conventional responses to any epidemic will be inadequate. He writes:

> A polity that is focused on chronic degenerative disease, that embraces cost control as the chief goal of health policy, and in which central authority is diminishing cannot address this epidemic as it has others of the recent past. . . . If the polity responds to AIDS as it has done since 1981, it is likely that the epidemic will be another incident in the gradual decline of collective responsibility for the human condition in the United States.[6]

It is difficult to evaluate this forceful argument, since historical experience is of limited applicability. Past epidemics, such as the influenza epidemic after World War I that killed 500,000 in the United States in one year, occurred in a society with many fewer resources. The response to the outbreak of Legionnaires disease that took twenty-nine lives in 1976 was prompt, despite interagency fumbling and infighting.[7] Had the cases begun doubling every six months, as was true of AIDS in the early stages, we believe that funds for research, prevention, and treatment would have poured forth for this new disease that affected middle-class visitors of convention centers, despite the state of the public health system. The response to the toxic shock syndrome was slow and barely adequate but much better, it seems to us, than the response to the AIDS epidemic.

The response of President Ford, the federal bureaucracy, and the drug industry to the swine flu epidemic bordered on the comical (had it not been for loss of life), but the comedy was partly the overresponse, not an underresponse. On the basis of only three cases of swine flu in a military camp, we proceeded to inoculate millions. The drug industry was late in producing the vaccine and demanded immunity from any suits claiming faulty vaccine quality. Dr. David Sencer was head of the CDC at the time. In contrast to his behavior much later when he was the New York City Health Commissioner denying an AIDS epidemic, at this time he

---

6. Fox, "AIDS and the American Health Polity," pp. 18, 26, 29.
7. Culliton, "Legion Fever."

ignored warnings that three cases do not an epidemic make and convinced President Ford that a supreme national effort was necessary. Twenty
or more deaths resulted from the vaccination program.[8]

The record, then, is mixed; we have done better in some cases, though
the cases are hardly comparable; we have many more resources to do
much better than we have had in the past, but in many respects, as noted
by Fox, we are more vulnerable now than before. Even though organizations in general and health care agencies in particular were prone to
failure, we will argue in the next chapter that more than a bureaucratic
bungle was involved in the case of AIDS.

THE REAGAN ADMINISTRATION: REDUCING PUBLIC SPENDING

A second reason for organizational failure in the AIDS crisis is
the Reagan administration's aversion to any increase in spending for
human services—or most governmental activities other than defense.
We count this as important because this resistance to what was called
"big government" occasionally overrode ideological considerations
and even interfered with life-saving efforts directed toward people for
whom there was widespread sympathy. For example, stopping the drug
trade would appear to be a natural endeavor for an administration that
embraces the "moral majority" groups, and domestic spending for appre-
hending drug dealers would seem to be a top priority. Yet funds for the
"war on drugs" were frequently cut on budgetary grounds. Similarly,
the race to develop superconductors following the breakthrough in high-
temperature superconductivity would appear to serve virtually every
legitimate goal of the administration, including increasing business
profits, increasing our defense, and improving economic growth and
competitiveness. The "crisis" had some of the overtones of the AIDS
crisis: researchers were raiding other programs in materials science to
work on the new developments for funds, few graduate students had
been attracted to the area before, and publicity was considerable. A

8. See Dutton, *Worse Than the Disease*.

large conference was held to announce the heavy commitment of the federal government, and many promises were made. One year later funding for the general area of materials science had not only not been increased but was cut by 20 percent. Graduate students stayed away for lack of funds, and the raids on other projects continued.[9] Japan and Europe surged ahead.

One final, deadly example from the AIDS experience. When an antibody blood test was finally available for screening the blood supply, Congress approved $8.4 million to make the test available to the blood banks. But the administration would not release the funds, though presumably it did not harbor any enmity toward hemophiliacs and the countless middle- and upper-class patients requiring transfusions, all at the risk of infection and death. Asked about the delay after several months, the administration would say only that the matter was "still under discussion."[10]

Thus, budget considerations may have played a sizable role in the response of the federal administration independent of the ideological and community pressures to "punish" HIV carriers. Shilts reports that the Office of Management and the Budget had no objections to the Secretary of Health and Human Services spending as much of the department's $6 billion budget on AIDS as she wished; she just could not have extra money for AIDS, so something else would have to be cut. Panem makes a similar observation.[11] In an administration that attempted each year to cut expenditures on health and human services, AIDS was not likely to get new money and would have a hard time displacing old programs. There was "tension among individual PHS agencies, the DHHS [Department of Health and Human Services], and Congress."[12] Financial considerations could have kept the blood industry from screening for hepatitis B (for the profit-making companies a 10 percent increase in cost could be important if it led to lower sales) and from jeopardizing

9. Mark Crawford, "Superconductor Funds Flat."

10. Shilts, *And the Band Played On*, p. 502.

11. Shilts, p. 288; Panem, *AIDS Bureaucracy*, pp. 80–81, 90–91.

12. Office of Technology Assessment, *Review of the Public Health Service's Response*, pp. 6–7.

the blood supply by asking high-risk persons not to donate. And, of course, the bathhouse owners would have ample reason not to post strong warnings in the houses or to close them. But we expect that had an epidemic broken out that affected, say, middle- and upper-class consumers of fine wine and liquor, congressional appropriations two or three times those made for AIDS would have been welcomed and quickly spent by the administration. [13]

THE IDEOLOGY OF THE "MORAL MAJORITY"

A third reason commonly cited to explain why government mishandled the AIDS epidemic is the alliance of the Reagan administration with those groups loosely labeled the "moral majority." AIDS victims are highly stigmatized; any administration would face obstacles in mobilizing government and private groups. But this administration was particularly beholden to the moral majority and thus particularly unenthusiastic about taking action. Conservative groups reportedly were successful in blocking educational programs and limiting counseling services; it is possible that they even blocked appropriations for research, education, and treatment programs.

Congress is less beholden to the conservative groups than the administration and was more responsive. The House and Senate consistently voted far more funds than the administration sought and threatened to go

13. Consider this fantasy: A rare mold appears in church organs and contaminates the congregations. Despite repeated warnings from church leaders and government officials, many churches insist upon staying open to accommodate their members, who prefer to risk the deadly mold infection than to risk damnation. The federal government commits $10 billion to research and organ sterilization despite the huge federal deficit, and the most talented researchers, sensing a Nobel prize, drop their other work to deal with this problem. The electronics industry institutes a crash program to create synthesizers that will mimic a wheezy organ. Passages are discovered in sacred texts that justify staying away from church, and the public schools are opened up for Saturday and Sunday services, thus persuading the faithful to give up their near-compulsive pattern and modify their risky behavior.

We have no doubt that despite the tendency to organizational failure, organizations and individuals will respond when certain majority values are in jeopardy.

to court when the administration refused to spend the allocations. A few members of Congress went to considerable lengths to increase funding for research, treatment, and education. While some of these were from northern California, where the gay vote is significant, others were not, and, most important, large majorities in both houses of Congress went along. Congressional appropriations have exceeded administration requests by 76 to 115 percent every year from 1983 to 1988.[14] But the response of state and local authorities (except in California and San Francisco) was far less positive. Indeed, one of the ironies of New York State politics is that liberal Democrat Governor Mario Cuomo, hardly beholden to the moral majority, threatened to veto AIDS bills that were overwhelmingly supported by the Republicans. Democratic Governor Michael Dukakis of Massachusetts was also quite reluctant to spend the monies the elected representatives offered.[15]

On the one hand, the influence of the moral majority, while undeniable, failed to stop Congress; on the other hand, some of those who were not subject to the moral majority in any substantial way held back their support. Government was not of a piece, even at the federal level, and funds, though inadequate according to the health agencies dealing with the epidemic, did appear. We can include this argument for failure by ideology with those of financial stringency and typical organizational failure: true but not sufficient.

It remains possible that the crisis in the health care sector is a true and sufficient reason for the weak response to the epidemic. The severely weakened state of the health care "system" in cities such as New York was sufficient to disable care and prevention programs. AIDS may have overloaded a precarious system to such an extent that unprecedented failures at the institutional and organizational level were ensured. We have no way of testing this "breakdown" thesis against the argument that AIDS is unique among health problems. To some degree they are not in conflict. But we feel that a crisis on the order of AIDS that affected nonstigmatized citizens would have been fought with more resources

14. General Accounting Office, *AIDS Prevention*.
15. Shilts, p. 559.

and less organizational denial, regardless of the state of the health system. In any case, our major concern is to explore the organizational response to AIDS; demonstrating that AIDS is a unique disease, as we shall try to do in the next chapter, completes the picture but is not essential to documenting the breakdown.

4   THE UNIQUE FEATURES OF AIDS

AIDS in America has two primary sources at present: unprotected anal intercourse, which is associated with gay male behavior and which probably accounts for the bulk of the existing cases nationwide; and intravenous drug injection with virus-contaminated needles, which is currently the major source of new cases and is likely to be the source of most cases within a few years.[1] Table 4-1 gives some of the recent statistics for the world, the United States, and New York City.

The characteristics of AIDS that make it unique among public health problems are best seen by contrasting AIDS with other health problems. Since it has appeared in epidemic form, it is appropriate to contrast it with potentially damaging *conditions*, such as infection by the polio virus; but since it involves activity patterns that can be deliberately changed, it can also be contrasted with the results of potentially damaging *behaviors*, such as compulsive eating or drinking. And since it involves sexual and drug habits, it can be contrasted with the problems caused by these potentially damaging behaviors *as they existed before AIDS*.

1. The other pathways for AIDS known today are transfusions with contaminated blood or blood products used by hemophiliacs, perinatal transmission from mother to fetus, heterosexual transmissions, and, extremely rare, unusual contact with the virus by health care or child care personnel. Though still small, the fastest growing group of AIDS cases is female partners of IVDUs and their babies.

Table 4-1. *Some basic statistics on the AIDS epidemic*

Persons with HIV	World: 5–10 million Africa: 3–4 million United States: 1–1.5 million[1]
AIDS cases in the United States	Cumulative, as of November 1989: 115,158[2]

Transmission
categories (U.S.)
	60% homosexual or bisexual male
	21% intravenous drug user
	  7% both homosexual or bisexual male and
	       intravenous drug user
	  5% heterosexual contact
	  2% recipient of blood transfusion
	  1% pediatric
	  1% hemophiliac
	  3% other

New cases (U.S.)	About 686 new cases were reported every week during 1989, as opposed to 618/week during 1988[3]
Deaths (U.S.)	As of November 1989: 68,441, or 60% of all cases[2]
Cases in New York City	Cumulative, as of November 1989: 23,066; active: 10,263[4]
Deaths (N.Y.C.)	As of November 1989: 12,803, or 56% of all cases[4]
Persons with HIV (N.Y.C.)	200,000[5]
Living situations for persons with AIDS (N.Y.C)	Hospitals: 1,531[6] Homeless in shelters: 1,000–2,000[7] City-subsidized apartments: 777[7] Municipal beds: 600[8] Other and unaccounted for: 1,479–2,479[9]
In New York and San Francisco	Over 50% of gay men have AIDS or HIV[10]

1. James Chin, "Current and Future Dimensions of the HIV/AIDS Pandemic," paper presented at the International Institute for Applied Systems Analysis (IIASA) Workshop in Budapest, Hungary, November 23–24, 1989, p. 26. CDC estimates for the end of 1987 range from 945,000 to 1.4 million in the United States, whereas Hudson Institute estimates range from 1.9 to 3.0 million. See "AIDS Virus Test in Midwest Indicated Low Infection Rate," *New York Times*, April 16, 1988; Philip M. Boffey, "Research Group Says AIDS Cases May Be Twice the U.S. Estimate," *New York Times*, August 20, 1988. The Hudson Institute reports that 200,000 to 500,000 non-IVDU heterosexuals are infected with the virus; CDC's estimate is 80,000 to 165,000.

2. Centers for Disease Control, *HIV/AIDS Surveillance Report*, December 1989, pp. 1–16.

3. Based on reported cases between December 1988 and November 1989 (for 1989), and December 1987 and November 1988 (for 1988).

4. New York City Department of Health AIDS Surveillance Unit, *AIDS Surveillance Update*, November 29, 1989.

5. Estimate down from a previous figure of 400,000. Bruce Lambert, "AIDS Count: Is the Quest for Precision on the Right Track?" *New York Times*, July 24, 1988.

6. Bruce Lambert, "Outlook Dim for Expanding Health Care," *New York Times*, April 5, 1988. Other estimates go up to 2,800 beds occupied by persons with AIDS.

7. Gina Kolata, "New York Shelters, a Last Stop for Hundreds of AIDS Patients," *New York Times*, April 4, 1988.

8. Figure is an estimate.

9. Number of New York City active cases as of April 1988 (6,387), less cases accounted for in the four previous categories.

10. Philip M. Boffey, "Spread of AIDS Abating, But Deaths Will Still Soar," *New York Times*, February 14, 1988.

INTENTIONAL BEHAVIOR

The important contrast with infectious diseases of the past, such as polio, swine flu, Legionnaires disease, and the more distant ones such as cholera, is that for these diseases changing one's behavior did not protect one from the disease. The 20 million worldwide victims of the influenza epidemic of 1918–19 (500,000 in the United States) could have done nothing to protect themselves. Even in the polio epidemic during the first half of this century, protective measures were limited to such things as public laws requiring children to remain indoors during the hottest days of the summer. (For a disease like tuberculosis, avoiding others with the disease is sufficient protection, but this is not possible for city dwellers, and especially the poor among them.)

We believe that the possibility of changing one's behavior to avoid infection is fundamental to understanding the response to AIDS. Once the information on AIDS is available, supermarket remedies will prevent infection for the great majority of those whose behavior puts them at risk of being exposed to HIV (that is, excluding cases of blood transfusion, use of blood products by hemophiliacs, and pediatric cases). It may be very difficult in some subcultures for a female partner to leave a man at risk of AIDS who refuses to use a condom, but it is possible. Because PWAs are seen as willing participants in the acts by which they became infected, they are held responsible for their infection, and concern over their civil liberties and care has been less compassionate than the concern shown for "the innocent." This has important consequences for charges of antihomosexual reactions to the AIDS crisis: even among people who are *not* antihomosexual, there are those who have been critical of the minority of gay men who continued to have unprotected anal sex with multiple partners after the risk was publicized.

DEGREES OF CULTURAL TOLERANCE OR HELP

There is a host of potentially damaging behaviors for which the damaged person is held accountable, so that in itself does not make AIDS unique. But we have widespread cultural tolerance for the most prevalent of these damaging behaviors, in contrast with the intolerance shown persons who have AIDS. Our society has evolved a culture of reasonable tolerance for, and offered some assistance in making behavioral changes to, those suffering from the widespread compulsions of smoking, overeating, gambling, and alcoholism. Despite the fact that these behaviors are seen as avoidable and self-inflicted, we have medical programs to deal with the symptoms and associated disabilities (such as cirrhosis of the liver caused by alcoholism or lung cancer caused by smoking) as well as programs to help change the (voluntary) behavior that caused the disorder. Public funds are available for these purposes, and their use is not considered controversial. We also find routine and substantial research on the etiology of many offending behaviors. And we find the disorders incorporated into a mildly stigmatizing but still tolerant and generally humorous folklore.

Most citizens, therefore, partake of the offending behaviors in mild degrees or have done so at some point in time. These people understand, and thus are more tolerant of, the problems of excess eating, alcohol, smoking, prescription drug abuse, and even gambling. The offending behavior is not strongly linked to class or minority status. The social costs—or externalities, as they are called—are tolerated even though they are borne by society at large or by persons who do not indulge in the behavior, through tax-supported medical costs, unemployment, early death, and in some cases the death of others (as in auto accidents) or the support of families that have been abandoned. This degree of tolerance is not extended to persons with AIDS (PWAs).[2]

It should be noted that there is nothing immutable or enduring about intolerance. Over time these behaviors may become more or less tolerated, associated more or less with stigmatized groups, seen as more or less involuntary. Marijuana smoking is not on our list because it is changing in status. It may achieve the social and legal tolerance that alcohol addiction has achieved, especially as society realizes that it is far less physically damaging than drinking or smoking legal substances and causes fewer deaths. It is possible that in time the lack of tolerance associated with AIDS will subside.

But tolerance is not extended to two other behaviorally related groups: users of illegal drugs and those who have contracted sexually transmitted diseases other than AIDS and prior to the appearance of AIDS. Both of these groups, however, can be distinguished from PWAs.

THE POSSIBILITY OF UNWITTING TRANSMISSION

Before AIDS, users of cocaine, heroin, and crack (though the last was not widespread until well after the appearance of AIDS) differed from today's IVDUs in that they could not transmit a fatal disease to others unwittingly or unknowingly. Hepatitis B and other nonfatal

2. Kagay, "Poll Finds Antipathy."

disorders might be transmitted through shared needles, but they are treatable diseases. Furthermore, the general public and public service workers did not fear picking up diseases from drug users unknowingly. (There was some fear among health care workers, especially surgeons, of getting hepatitis B from drug addicts, but there is now a vaccine.) This dimension of the disease of AIDS is particularly menacing as the latency period of the disease—the time it takes for it to manifest itself in disorders—is discovered to be longer and longer, up to eight to ten years at the present. Surveys indicate that 25 percent of the population think the disease can be spread by coughing.[3] Health care workers fear that a seropositive patient who is not diagnosed as having AIDS may transmit it in fairly casual ways. Both beliefs are unfounded, of course, but AIDS is unusual in this respect. Unwitting transmission of the virus can occur, however, through sharing unsterilized needles, through homosexual or heterosexual contacts, and through the use of contaminated blood.

If a threatening condition can be transmitted unknowingly and unwittingly from a human carrier to another human, it will be treated differently than if the source were a virus generated by swine, mold, or other nonhuman agents. There is an element of menace or threat in person-to-person transmission. If, in addition, there is a long latency period during which carriers may not even know that they can transmit the disease, and still worse, if they do know but wish to disguise the fact, the potentially damaging condition is feared even more. We would view alcoholism or coke sniffing with far more alarm if the damaging physical consequences of cirrhosis or immune-system suppression could be transmitted to another person by the alcoholic or coke user. The tentative findings about passive smoking probably had a great deal to do with antismoking legislation; when it was demonstrated that breathing another's smoke was a health danger, smoking was seen as a greater menace.

The transmission problem becomes a civil liberties issue. Though we have legislation restricting the freedom of those with active tuberculosis and those with syphilis to infect others, and some seek similar laws regarding those with HIV infection, the enforcement of such legislation

3. Blendon and Donelan, "Discrimination against People with AIDS."

jeopardizes civil rights. By avoiding detection the HIV-seropositive person can enjoy normal civil rights (and thus not be fired, lose insurance coverage, be denied access to housing or public schools); these rights could easily disappear if the seropositive condition is detected. Thus many in high-risk groups resist taking the HIV-antibody test lest they lose their jobs, insurance, housing, and freedom of movement.[4]

SEXUAL AND OTHER STIGMAS

Sexually transmitted diseases that result from casual or commercial sex, and especially from unprotected anal sex, partake of all the characteristics we've mentioned. They are due to changeable behavior, there is little or no cultural tolerance available for them, and they can be transmitted unknowingly. But unprotected anal sex is further characterized by the special sexual stigma attached to it, either as an "unnatural act" among heterosexuals or as a homosexual act. We know almost nothing about the prevalence of anal intercourse among heterosexuals; it is a very private behavior that leaves no "markers." It is the category of male homosexual acts that is the most relevant to AIDS. It was stigmatizing even before AIDS and probably has become even more so since AIDS. Though the stigma is different from that associated with the unsterilized injection of drugs once AIDS appeared upon the scene, we will treat both stigmas together.

Once AIDS came on the scene, male homosexuals and IVDUs experienced a societal reaction that goes beyond the absence of cultural tolerance or help and the fear of transmission: gay men faced a homophobia grown more intense, and IVDUs met with a disapproval now mixed with fear and, often, racism. Prior to the appearance of AIDS, there were many middle-class and working-class IVDUs who, as long as they were not gay men or black or Hispanic, were not stigmatized. With the appearance of AIDS, we would argue, white heterosexual drug abusers are

4. For a good, brief discussion of the dangers of compulsory testing, see Weiss and Thier, "HIV Testing Is the Answer—What's the Question?" The authors are from the Institute of Medicine of the National Academy of Sciences.

stigmatized; they leave a category with only two strikes against it—disapproval of the act itself, and the fact that the act is seen as voluntary—and move to one with two additional strikes: the fear that the disease may unknowingly or secretly be transmitted, and the association of the disease with two stigmatized groups—homosexual men and impoverished blacks and Hispanics.

Stigmatization involves social isolation, such that people have to leave their normal living situation and live alone or with others in the same plight; isolation at the workplace or other public places; fear of job loss even if the condition does not affect job performance; possible loss of social entitlements such as health care, social security, unemployment insurance, commercial insurance, and access to public housing; a low priority in terms of government funding for research, treatment, and education and, also important, extensive controversy over that funding; and lack of normal access to resources for coping with problems (private charity, churches, short-term credit, social clubs, and so on).

Some of the stigma associated with AIDS is transferred to another group: hemophiliacs. As we shall note in Chapter 6, the fact that hemophiliacs were dying of AIDS in large numbers as a result of contaminated blood products that they needed meant that the New York Chapter of the National Hemophilia Foundation began to lose volunteer fund raisers and board members, who did not want to be associated with the stigmatized condition. Hemophiliacs with AIDS do not share all the other negative factors we have been considering. Their illness was not due to any behavior that they could change. By and large, cultural tolerance and help were still available, though they were diminished, even though unwitting transmission was possible. (It is also possible that some of the stigma associated with AIDS is being transferred to those heterosexuals who have multiple casual sexual encounters, though there is no documented evidence of this.)

The interaction of mysterious diseases and stigmatized populations is dramatically drawn in Zachary Gussow's book *Leprosy, Racism, and Public Health*.[5] Leprosy is a very old disease, but its association with

5. Gussow, "Social Policy and Chronic Disease Control," in *Leprosy, Racism, and Public Health*.

stigma has been neither continuous nor universal. Westerners in the nineteenth century often associated the disease with inferior peoples as they came across it in their colonial empires, and fear of leprosy was used to limit immigration to the United States in the late nineteenth and early twentieth centuries. Many Americans, already persuaded of racist beliefs, found it easy to link the disease with hated foreign groups, especially the Chinese (who were called the "Yellow Peril" because of the disease). The handful of lepers in the United States were isolated and contained in Louisiana.

In Norway, however, where the disease was hyperendemic among the rural poor, there was little racism in the nation and no racial categories with which to link the disease. The government established clinics and treatment centers and sponsored the basic research that led to identification of the infectious agent by Armauer Hansen. Even though Hansen called for isolation of lepers, because it was still unclear how infectious the disease was, the Norwegian government resisted; it continued to sponsor research and emphasize a strictly medical approach. In our terms, the fact that Norwegians, rather than people of another race or ethnicity, had the disease, even though they were poor, meant that there was only a low hurdle in the way of "medicalizing" the disease for the government to overcome. This hurdle was readily overcome because there was, in so homogeneous a culture, more tolerance of poverty. In the United States and other nations, the presence of racism in general and the concentration of leprosy (Hansen's disease, it is now called) among racial groups meant that the government and private health authorities had a high hurdle to overcome. They did not succeed, and the disease was, in contrast, "moralized." It seems to be so with AIDS in the United States as compared with AIDS in some European countries.

UNUSUAL SOCIAL AND MEDICAL DISABILITIES

Finally, persons with AIDS are subject to a long list of unusual social and medical disabilities. While a few of these may be shared with the other groups we have been considering—victims of other infections diseases, of compulsions, drug abuse before AIDS, and sexually transmitted diseases—AIDS appears to be unique in exhibiting them all.

The virus is still changing and is deceptive in its invasion of the body; no vaccines or cures are currently available, and palliatives are limited to a few drugs, especially AZT; the care is very expensive; the course of the disease is long and painful and disfiguring; there is a potential risk to health care workers; there is an unfounded but widespread fear of contamination through casual contact, such as sharing tools or kitchen or toilet facilities; the hospital system is being overwhelmed by AIDS patients, and there is an acute shortage of nurses, orderlies, and other care personnel; and death appears to be certain (though we have not been into the epidemic long enough to know for sure).

THE PERIL, THE STIGMA, AND THE COST

Figure 4-1 summarizes our discussion and highlights the special character of AIDS. It emphasizes that PWAs suffer from *all* of the problems that may complicate effective social response to a disease. Our scale is cumulative for the most part. In the public view, the infection is caused by behavior that could have been avoided, thus making PWAs responsible for their plight even if they were uninformed of the consequences of the behavior. Even if the behavior that led to AIDS is thought to be compulsive, as in the case of drug addiction, it is not given the tolerance of compulsive smoking, drinking, eating, or gambling. Because HIV may be carried by a person for a long time before it is discovered, the person may infect others unwittingly; when they learn of their condition they are reluctant to disclose it or even seek help because their civil liberties will be curtailed when they most need them. IVDUs are violating the law, and conservative elements of our society are seeking to make homosexual behavior illegal (it already is in about half of the states, and there have been a few prosecutions) and to criminalize some behaviors of PWAs. The stigmas are very pronounced. Finally, the medical aspects are extreme; treatment is expensive and prolonged, and the disease is debilitating and fatal.

These elements are not only cumulative but are interactive for PWAs and the risk groups they come from. There is a "system effect" in that failures in one part of the social system interact with failures in another.

Figure 4-1. *Features of a disease or behavior that lessen tolerance or increase fear of the disease or behavior*

Potentially damaging conditions or behavior	Due to changeable behavior	Little or no cultural tolerance or help	Possibility of unwitting transmission	Sexual or other stigma	Unusual social or medical aspects*
Before AIDS					
Infectious diseases Polio, swine flu, Legionnaires disease	no	no	no	no	no
Widespread compulsions Smoking, obesity, gambling, alcoholism	yes	no	no	no	no
Drugs IV injection, coke, sniff, crack	yes	yes	no	no	no
Sexually transmitted diseases					
Casual/commercial sex	yes	yes	yes	no	no
Unprotected anal sex	yes	yes	yes	yes	no
Coupled with AIDS					
Hemophilia	no	partial	yes	partial	yes
Heterosexual casual contact	yes	no	yes	partial	yes
IV unsterilized injection	yes	yes	yes	yes	yes
Unprotected homosexual sex Anal intercourse, semen injection	yes	yes	yes	yes	yes

* Social: civil liberties dilemmas; screening; quarantine. Medical: changing virus; no vaccines or cures or palliative; expensive care; bed and nurse shortage; long, painful dying; fatal.

For example, the possibility of changing a risky behavior aggravates the stigma attached to that behavior. Even if homosexuality is accepted, the changeable-behavior dimension places gay men in the IVDU category —people may be accepting of the sexual preference but still hold gay men accountable for not taking precautions. Medical aspects such as fear of contamination reinforce the cultural isolation and intolerance. The minority status of many PWAs means that few resources are allotted in the community for care and prevention.

In contrast to the blacks and Hispanics, the white homosexual population is fairly affluent and politically sophisticated, and it has its own community. The gay male population has been very effective, especially in San Francisco, in developing resources, securing an immense amount of volunteer labor, and gaining civil liberties protection. In New York City, it has organized an extremely effective education and self-help group, the Gay Men's Health Crisis, which constituted the only substantial response to the epidemic for four years. Affluence and political sophistication, however, have not been able to make up for the deficits of cultural intolerance and sexual stigmatization and the debilitating medical aspects of AIDS.

If we add to the characteristics of the AIDS epidemic shown in Figure 4-1 the other conditions we have detailed—organizational ineffectiveness and weakness of the public health sector, the economic concerns of the Reagan administration, and the administration's alliance with the moral majority—we can begin to see why the AIDS epidemic is overwhelming the normal defenses of organizations.

The problems might be summarized as threefold: peril, stigma, and cost. The *peril*, or threat, is to the rest of the population as the disease spreads beyond IVDUs and gay men. (As it is checked by drugs such as AZT and as the more privileged classes are better educated, the disease will be "redlined" and the peril for the general public will decrease.) The *stigma* is attached to the disease because it affects primarily gay men and IVDUs. The *financial* burden is on government, private care providers, and insurance companies. A fourth problem, that of *system effects*, concerns the unexpected interaction of failures. Each individual failure in housing, employment discrimination, hospital bed shortages, rise in syphilis, and so on might be considered the particular problem of the appropriate authority (housing authority, employment agency, hospital commission, public health agencies). But if, as we shall see, the bed shortage means that some patients without housing will be discharged with a false diagnosis in order to free up a bed, and then are sexually assaulted in a poorly supervised shelter, possibly spreading the virus to the aggressor, we have an unanticipated "systems effect." We shall discover several in the coming chapters.

To draw out the consequences of the special nature of AIDS, we will present our findings on the responses of New York State and New York City organizations to the crisis in more detail; our work is based on interviews with the heads, or assistant heads, of some sixty-five organizations or units in New York City.[6]

6. Interviews were open-ended and notes were taken. We used a "snowball" sample; that is, we scanned the literature and asked respondents for the names of organizations that were either providing direct care for PWAs or coordinating, planning, or overseeing such care. Many organizations or units of organizations repeatedly canceled the interviews or turned us down outright. The first wave of interviews took place between August and December 1987; further interviews took place in the spring and summer of 1988. About one-quarter of all completed interviews were judged to be noncooperative or hostile, an unprecedented degree of resistance in the experience of the senior author, who has conducted interview studies in a variety of public and private organizations for three decades.

5 THE CRISIS IN NEW YORK

AIDS came to a city particularly ill prepared to cope with it. Experts writing in the late 1970s routinely discussed the fragmentation of New York's health care sector and its exploding costs.[1] Fragmentation of both health care and health insurance is characteristic of the United States as compared with other industrialized societies, but within the United States, the degree of fragmentation in New York sets it apart from other cities and states. The impact of any health crisis is bound to be greater in New York City than in any other American city. For instance, it is generally agreed that the response to the AIDS epidemic was faster and better coordinated in San Francisco than in New York. But San Francisco has a small, manageable health care industry consisting of just one acute-care municipal hospital, thirteen private and voluntary hospitals, and one medical school. The health care sector in New York, a city six times as large, includes eleven municipal hospitals, seventy private and voluntary hospitals, and seven medical schools. In San Francisco the health director can coordinate medical affairs across the city. He or she supervises public health facilities, including mental health care, drug-abuse programs, the municipal hospitals, and the nursing home services. In New York these are all run by separate agencies; any

1. See, for example, Rossman and Pomrinse, "New York City"; and Pomrinse, Allen, and Rossman, "Health Care in a Big City."

coordination has to come from the mayor, but the mayor's position is not a strong one. Thus, the scale and complexity of New York's health care sector far exceed those of San Francisco's.[2]

Health care costs were rising faster in New York than in other American cities, at least until the mid-1970s. By then, annual per capita expenditures on health were $885, as opposed to the national average of $514.[3] Whereas in 1966 public and private expenditures on health accounted for 8 percent of the personal income of New Yorkers, the proportion reached 14 percent in 1975.[4]

New York not only spends more on health than other cities, but a larger part of health expenditures is financed publicly by the city government, and the federal contribution to New York City's health care bill is less than it is elsewhere.[5] It did not help matters that during the 1970s both New York City and New York State had greater budget deficits than most other cities and states. Thus, the city appeared to be at fiscal risk when AIDS arrived in 1982. We were routinely reminded of these problems, and especially of the deficits in the late 1970s, when we interviewed city and state agencies. But the 1980s were boom years for New York City,[6] and the city's largesse with tax rebates and municipal corruption have been frequently noted. In addition, city hospitals were eliminating beds in the 1980s even as the growing AIDS burden demanded more.

Since 1978 many national health care experts have addressed the problems of rising costs and sinking performance from a rationalist, market-oriented, short-term perspective. One diagnosis has been

2. Some studies suggest that this complexity hampers New York City's effort, and we are sure it does. But it is probably more important that the city has consistently spent less on AIDS than San Francisco has. Arno and Hughes, "Local Policy Responses."
3. Rossman and Pomrinse, "New York City," p. 53.
4. Piore, Lieberman, and Linnane, "Public Expenditures and Private Control?," especially p. 88.
5. Pomrinse, Allen, and Rossman, "Health Care in a Big City," p. 282; Piore, Lieberman, and Linnane, "Public Expenditures and Private Control?"
6. Renshaw, Trott, and Friedenberg, "Gross State Product by Industry, 1963–1986."

overcapacity—underutilized beds—in cities as the suburbs built their own hospitals. For example, in 1978 some health care experts reported that in New York City "from 4,000 to 5,000 hospital beds should be considered 'surplus'."[7] Though they could hardly have foreseen the wave of infectious hospitalization that was to take place later in the 1980s, these experts failed to prepare for the widely predicted shift from a preponderance of short-term acute patients to a greater proportion of patients needing long-term chronic care. (The acutely ill went to the suburbs while the chronic patients stayed in the city.) Instead, the experts were disposed to emphasize life-style changes to improve the health of the community and cost-containment mechanisms to cut costs. The logic was that if we could stop smoking and drinking and overeating, hospital beds could be removed. The perspective of the 1950s and 1960s, which had linked public health problems to infectious agents, unequal access to preventive and health care resources, and environmental pollution, was set aside.[8]

Experts and policymakers could not possibly have foreseen the coming of the AIDS epidemic in its full scale until about 1983, when New York City passed the symbolic barrier of 1,000 reported cases. But even after 1986 we find, on a national as well as a city basis, failures to recognize the potential spread of AIDS and the quantity and quality of health services needed. Those failures were especially important and persistent in New York City. Writing in the *New England Journal of Medicine*, David Weinberg and Henry Murray dryly note: "Using a mathematical model, the New York City Health Department suggested in early 1987 that 8,300 new cases would be diagnosed in 1991. Using national data collected since 1981, the Centers for Disease Control (CDC) put the figure at about 20,000 cases in New York City," an estimate two and a half times as large.[9] Since the city's health department had both competent experts and the CDC data, this discrepancy suggests that political pressures were at work. Another estimate, made by the Interagency Task Force on AIDS a year later (May 1988), increased the

7. Rossman and Pomrinse, "New York City," p. 69.
8. Fox, "AIDS and the American Health Polity."
9. Weinberg and Murray, "Coping with AIDS."

city's likely number of new cases for 1991 to "between 7,876 and 11,232."[10] And even CDC figures might well be an underestimate of the scope of the epidemic; the Hudson Institute, a private research organization, estimated that the CDC projections for 1991 reflected only half the number of persons believed to be infected with the virus at present.[11] The General Accounting Office also warned that "only about two-thirds of all persons with AIDS and other fatal HIV-related illnesses were captured in the data underlying existing national forecasts."[12] Moreover, "the lag time between diagnosis and report to [New York City's] Department of Health is usually under six months, but has been as long as 24 months."[13]

Incredibly, according to one study, "in late 1986 and early 1987, in response to a range of regulatory and economic pressures, the city's hospitals closed approximately 1,800 inpatient beds," about 5 percent of total capacity.[14] It is worth mentioning that the number of hospital patient-days associated with AIDS was growing at an annual rate of 20–25 percent at this time. Less than three years later, business elites raised the alarm concerning the consequences of the bed shortage.

Unfortunately, the highest officials of the city and state continued to deny the need for additional facilities and services. Mayor Koch's health budgets were criticized in late 1988 and in 1989 for "jeopardizing patient care by failing to meet the crises of hospital overcrowding and the AIDS epidemic" in spite of the recommendations made by the Interagency Task Force on AIDS, a body never accused of being pessimistic, let alone hysterical.[15] There were warnings from several sources going back to 1987 of a collapse or "systemic failure" of the health care sector due to the lack of primary and preventive care, long-term facilities, home

10. Interagency Task Force on AIDS, *New York City Strategic Plan for AIDS*, Executive Summary, p. 1, and fig. 3.
11. Philip M. Boffey, "Research Group Says AIDS Cases May Be Twice the U.S. Estimate."
12. "Forecasts of AIDS Fall Short."
13. Aids Surveillance Unit, *AIDS Surveillance Update*, p. 3.
14. Bigel Institute, *New York City's Hospital Occupancy Crisis*.
15. Lambert, "Debate Swirls over Cuts."

care, drug treatment, and universal insurance. The warnings escalated
in 1988 and 1989.[16] The city tried to increase the financial commitment
of the state and federal governments, but state-run hospitals added less
than a third of the 500 new beds planned for 1988. State legislators
were "frustrated and angry" because "the Governor talks about how
much he's increasing funding, but he's sitting on a big chunk of what
was appropriated last year. The Legislature fought to get it in, and he's
in effect impounding it," said the state AIDS Council in a report.[17] The
Bush administration does not seem to be willing to increase, or even to
maintain, its share of the burden; it proposed a federal health care budget in 1989 that would cut funds available to New York City's hospitals
by at least $200 million.[18]

Even health care professionals and administrators — in opposing camps
on most issues — have recently agreed to criticize a cutback in city and
state health coverage programs in view of the fact that fully a quarter of
the population remains uninsured.[19] Critics have been proposing various
remedies for the health care problems posed by AIDS, such as the establishment of a large hospital dedicated to AIDS, the development of a
flexible system of extended out-of-hospital care, and the expansion of
methadone treatment programs for IVDUs.[20] Progress toward any of
those solutions has been slow or nonexistent, despite press releases about
a few facilities or beds here or there. But where facilities or beds finally
became available they remained unused because of the staggering difficulty in hiring new staff, especially nurses.[21] Following the dire warnings
of loss of jobs in business and industry because of the hospital-bed
shortage and a "Calcutta" scene in the city, Mayor Koch announced in
May 1989 that he would seek $40 million more for AIDS, but those

16. French, "Hospitals Overwhelmed"; Lambert, "Flaws in Health Care System
Emerge."
17. Lambert, "State AIDS Council Attacks Cuomo over Delays."
18. Lambert, "Cuomo Sets AIDS Plan"; May, "Hospitals Take Budget Woes to
Congress."
19. French, "New York Health Care Failure Charged"; French, "Unlikely Coalition Fights Cut"; Verhovek, "Cuomo Is Being Fought on Medicaid Cuts."
20. Weinberg and Murray, "Coping with AIDS," pp. 1471–1472. See also Lambert, "State AIDS Council Attacks Cuomo over Delays."
21. Okun, "Lack of Nurses Impedes New York AIDS Care."

familiar with his past pledges remained skeptical. Richard Dunne, executive director of the Gay Men's Health Crisis, applauded the extension of eligibility to those who were suffering from AIDS-related disorders but who did not quite meet the stringent definition of the CDC. But as for the plans for services and housing, he said, "We've had press conferences about assessment centers and housing going back years that never quite make it."[22]

Policymakers may be charged not only with failing to provide sufficient health care facilities, services, and professionals but also with underestimating the implications of the spread of AIDS among the homeless and the very poor. In fact, being poor and addicted to IV drugs increases both the likelihood of AIDS infection and the unlikelihood of appropriate health care. According to federal standards, the proportion of people below the poverty level in New York City rose over 50 percent in a decade, from 15 percent in 1975 to 24 percent in 1984, and is still increasing.[23] The reasons behind the steep increase lie in the deinstitutionalization of the chronically mentally ill, the rise of unemployment in the inner city, the discontinuation of welfare programs, and the conversion of low-rent housing into expensive condominiums and office space. Health officials seem to be downplaying the potential consequences of the "process of pauperization" as well as of increasing infection rates among IVDUs.

It has not helped the city that a resurgence of conservative views coincided with the AIDS epidemic. Conservatives say that government is too big, that it is unable to pay for what it does, and that what it does in its welfare programs is illegitimate anyway because it interferes with economic vitality. This point of view has complicated the handling of a full-scale epidemic such as AIDS.[24]

These variables, although they indicate serious problems, seem insufficient to explain the recurrent miscalculations and denials of the long-term nature of the epidemic. A more detailed account of the role played by

22. Lambert, "Koch to Seek $40 Million."
23. Imperato, "New York's Homeless."
24. For a valuable account of recent criticisms of the health care sector and of the welfare state in the United States, see Marmor, "American Medical Policy and the 'Crisis' of the Welfare State."

organizational actors may illuminate the factors associated with New York City's failure to respond promptly and adequately to the AIDS crisis.

Although we focus upon New York City, we should note that few other cities seem to be doing well. In most respects, for example, New York has done more than Philadelphia, though New Yorkers should take neither pride nor comfort in that.

In 1988 the Philadelphia Commission on AIDS released a report of a one-year study. It was critical of the established sectors of the community, namely business, religion, the media, health care institutions, and state and local government, for their "lagging leadership . . . poor funding . . . persistent prejudice and discrimination . . . and lack of coordinated programs of education, outreach, social services, or health care." In terms of total expenditures on diagnosed cases of AIDS, Philadelphia ranked thirty-sixth among cities, though it was ninth in the number of reported cases. The city allocated only $287 per case, while New York was spending $3,112 per case. (Hospital costs alone average $140,000 for each AIDS patient.) The six medical schools were judged to have made an "insufficient" response to AIDS. The city council voted only $70,000 for AIDS in 1987, though it increased the amount to $5 million in 1988. The inevitable coordinating office was created to oversee AIDS programs, but there were few programs.

As might be expected, the report found that for "the first seven years of the AIDS epidemic, virtually all human services for persons with AIDS in Philadelphia were provided by [grass-roots groups] operating on shoestring budgets and relying primarily on volunteers." Prior to the winter of 1988 these community-based organizations "also provided nearly all AIDS education to high risk groups."[25]

THE INITIAL RESPONSE

When New York State and City confronted the AIDS crisis in the early 1980s, most officials knew that the disease would be very expensive and that it affected gay men, was spreading rapidly, and might

25. Philadelphia Commission on AIDS, *Report to the Community*, p. 112.

spread into the general population. The reported cases initially were overwhelmingly among the highly active male homosexual population, and it was the gay community that pressured state and local authorities to take action in education, care, and research starting in 1982. Yet the exclusive focus on the gay population is puzzling. It was known from the start that IVDUs were at risk, and there were an estimated 200,000 of them in New York City. At least by May 1983, if not well before then, medical experts had warned New York State legislators that incidence among IVDUs and gay males was doubling every six months and would reach epidemic proportions.[26]

In addition to the warnings from medical experts, evidence of AIDS in the communities most affected by drug use was available from state and city agencies. The New York State Division of Substance Abuse was very well organized (even though, unlike some gay groups, the drug users were not), and it had methadone clinics and other drug treatment centers in place well before AIDS. The programs enrolled only a tiny fraction of the addicts, but that was enough to indicate the growing number of cases. The Substance Abuse Division, tiny and underfunded as it was, had many routes into the minority community; but like most organizations, it virtually ignored the problem for the first few years. Its mandate was to fight substance abuse, not the disease that was killing the abusers. Education programs among IVDUs would have been very difficult at that time, and still are, but almost any attempt would have been worth making when cases were known to be doubling every six months.[27]

Quite possibly the explanation for the emphasis on gay men has "structural" sources other than their political organization and the orientation of the Substance Abuse Division. Gerald Oppenheimer, in a thoughtful paper on the "epidemiological construction of AIDS," notes that in stud-

26. Ronald Sullivan, "Experts Testify."

27. Nick Freudenberg notes in his review of Shilts's *And the Band Played On* that drug users and minorities in general are barely mentioned in that otherwise quite exhaustive book. It is true, but it was true of virtually everyone writing on or working in the area until about 1986. The IVDUs were there in large numbers, and their growth could be anticipated, but they were invisible. Freudenberg, "Historical Omissions."

ies of the distribution of patients or the epidemiology of the disease in 1982 and 1983, heterosexual patients, particularly drug users and their sexual partners, were significantly underrepresented. Instead, the literature emphasized gay men's life-style. Even the *Journal of the American Medical Association* asked as early as 1982 why, if life-style was the key to the transmission of AIDS, there were so many cases of heterosexual men, women, and hemophiliacs with AIDS. The first significant attention to heterosexual risk groups began in 1984 with a series of papers by Don C. Des Jarlais, Samuel R. Friedman, and their colleagues in the State Division of Substance Abuse.

Oppenheimer argues that the reasons for the neglect of heterosexual IVDUs was organizational more than cultural. The experts on intravenous drug use at the National Institute of Drug Abuse (NIDA) were concerned with addiction but not with diseases associated with it, such as hepatitis B or endocarditis, which were endemic and even epidemic in the drug-using population. These diseases were studied by other federal organizations in the National Institutes of Health, ones not concerned with addiction. The Centers for Disease Control had no experience with the population that uses drugs, and of the small number of research subjects with AIDS initially available, the majority were gay men. One cultural matter that may have been influential, Oppenheimer notes, is that drug addicts are seen as of even less social consequence than gay men.[28]

It wasn't until about 1988 that the IVDUs and the gay male populations received parity in concern in New York City, as the number of drug-related cases steadily grew and the connection with prostitution and infants with HIV became more obvious. In 1988, perhaps as a result of this, New York City made a sweeping change in its estimate of the size of the two populations. The estimated number of IVDUs remained at 200,000, but the estimated number of homosexual males was cut fivefold, from 500,000 to 100,000. ("I know at least 100,000 myself!" one gay activist said in mock astonishment.) The latter estimate was based on decades-old Kinsey studies and extrapolations from data from

28. Gerald M. Oppenheimer, "In the Eye of the Storm."

San Francisco, which were more reliable than those of New York City. Both the gay male population and the IVDUs were still estimated to have an infection rate of 50 percent. Thus the "problem" was cut in half; the estimate of the number of gay and bisexual men and IVDUs with HIV in New York City went from 350,000 to 150,000, so the estimate of the *total* number of people infected in New York City went from 400,000 to 200,000.

As might be anticipated, gay activists protested that this cut was made to justify the low level of funding, but the new New York City Health Commissioner, Dr. Stephen Joseph, denied it. And, indeed, 1988 did see a substantial increase in funding. ("Medicine," Dr. Joseph was quoted as saying in connection with the fivefold reduction, "is a science, albeit an inexact one.")[29] Subsequent evidence, scanty though it is, suggests that some reduction was in order. But perhaps the most important observation is that by 1988 the city was finally beginning to think of the policy implications of the distribution of cases. The two major groups, gay men and IVDUs, would require different services and educational tactics, and they interacted in different ways with the abundant social and political problems.

Through most of the epidemic so far, however, the preoccupation has been with the largest group, gay men. It took a long time for health authorities to do more than just react to political pressures from the gay activists, the moral majority and the Catholic Church, minority politicians, and others who were defining the problem as gay-related. Thus, most of our discussion of the initial years will concern the response to the crisis in the male homosexual population rather than the minority IVDU population, which remained invisible, or was kept invisible, for so long.

Both the state and the city were slow to respond even to the deaths among homosexual men. San Francisco, with far fewer cases, was spending $4 million of its own money in 1983, when New York City was just making its first appropriations.[30] The Republican governor of California

29. Lambert, "Halving of Estimate on AIDS Is Raising Doubts."
30. Shilts, *And the Band Played On*, p. 400. Only 3 percent of the few community-based services in New York City in 1984 were financed by the city, whereas in San

made state funds available in 1982.[31] It was not until August 1983 that New York State made its first substantial move, the establishment of the Aids Institute (AI) with a small appropriation. In New York City, with 45 percent of the nation's AIDS cases, an Interagency AIDS Task Force was set up in the fall of 1982, but it was not charged with either program or fiscal responsibility. The next official response did not occur until March 9, 1983, and it was a curious organizational one. Two days before, gay activist Larry Kramer had published a blistering piece, "1,112 and Counting," in a gay newspaper the *New York Native*; widely attacked and discussed, it accused the mayor of inaction and of refusing to see gay leaders. Perhaps in response, two days later Mayor Koch set up an Office of Gay and Lesbian Health Concerns, a puzzling title since the disease had a name, affected male homosexuals and drug users and not lesbians, and was something more than a "health concern" since it was killing its victims. The office was headed by a prominent gay physician and advisor to the mayor, who shared leadership duties with a prominent lesbian.

It is not clear to us what the Office of Gay and Lesbian Health Concerns did regarding the AIDS crisis except to receive inquiries from the frantic members of the gay community. Its director did, however, take a strong stand opposing the closing of the bathhouses. When he claimed that he was not going to tell gay men how to have sex, he refused to do precisely what was needed in those early days of rapid spread. The director resigned a year and a half later, and the office seems to have faded, though it still exists. It was overrun by the rapid rise in cases and deaths, and the activity shifted to existing institutions that had to deal with the cases—the hospitals, prisons, drug programs, and the housing office.

At the Interagency AIDS Task Force, representatives from these various agencies talked about the need for education, hospice beds, nurses, and planning for future hospital beds. In September 1984, task force member Arthur Felson reported to the group about its accomplishments

Francisco the three largest programs received 62 percent of their funding from the city. See Lee and Arno, "AIDS and Health Policy," p. 15.

31. Arno and Hughes, "Local Policy Responses," p. 269.

over two years. As Shilts reports: "By Felson's count, the task force had discussed the problem of housing for AIDS patients sixteen times, the lack of any active surveillance in the city fourteen times, and the need for home health care eight times, all without any resulting moves by the city government." The Health Commissioner (at that time David Sencer) acknowledged the problem and promised to form another task force.[32]

THE AIDS INSTITUTE

The New York State AIDS Institute (AI) was not overrun by events as the mayor's Office of Gay and Lesbian Health Concerns was, and it prospers today, its budget increasing substantially every year and the scope of its activities expanding. It was placed in the State Department of Health in 1983, initially under an epidemiology office. The epidemiology of the virus was a paramount concern at the time and was the most well researched aspect of the epidemic. (Curiously enough, in 1983 one of the institute's leaders denied that there was an epidemic, since "only" about one in 1,000 gay men appeared to have the virus. About 1,200 cases of AIDS had been reported in New York City by then, 3,000 nationwide, and 1,283 of these had died.)[33] Now the institute is of equal rank with the epidemiology office and reports to the Director of Community Health, who in turn reports to the Health Commissioner. The institute was lauded in a George Washington University research project as an innovative model of a centralized response to the epidemic.[34] It was difficult for us in 1988 to determine the size of the staff concerned primarily with New York City (or even of the whole institute), but it appeared to be only four or five people. The fiscal 1987–88 budget for AI was some $16 million. The AI represents the state's primary response to the crisis.

We heard two stories about the AI in particular and the city and state

---

32. Shilts, p. 484.
33. Shilts, pp. 400, 401. Health Commissioner Sencer denied an epidemic as late as 1985. Ibid., p. 533.
34. Intergovernmental Health Policy Project, *Assessing the Problem*, p. 1–17.

response in general from a variety of respondents, and they reflected the inescapable dilemmas of centralization or decentralization, and of politics and techniques. Both are worth detailing in view of the available evidence, since they highlight the distinctive nature of the epidemic —the role of peril, stigma, and, of course, finances. The first is a cynical interpretation by "inside dopesters" and bitter community-group personnel. It stresses that AI was a *centralized*, program-specific attempt by the state to segregate the problem, "buy off" the gay population, spend as little money as possible, and ignore the minority and drug populations entirely. A decentralized response, in this view, would have been to increase the budget of various state and local bureaus—housing, education, corrections, community health services—to allow them to develop the appropriate programs for whoever the disease struck. This would medicalize rather than politicize the disease; it would be treated as special only in the amount of extra resources necessary.

The second interpretation is by personnel at the AIDS Institute itself. It stresses high uncertainty about the scope of the problem, the rationality and prudence of the responses of the governor down to the mayor, and the enormous obstacles to involving the minority community and the IVDUs. A centralized response was necessary because the disease was new and hit specific groups in the population, this story goes, and existing facilities were not prepared for it.

Both stories have their virtues and faults, and we suspect that both are too "rational" and too "intentional" as accounts. That is, much of what happened just happened as the health system and the political system stumbled along with an unusual amount of uncertainty, misinformation, fear, and possibly some loathing. There may have been little explicit planning and strategy, and respondents would be telling the "truth" if they said they did not intend to segregate the cases, protect the governor at the expense of the sick, and so on. But, given the political overtones of AIDS as a moralized disease and the incoherence of the health system, it is not surprising that an adequate response that utilized existing facilities in a coordinated way to deal with both the gay male and the IVDU and minority populations was not forthcoming.[35]

35. This judgment reflects an organizational perspective that goes under such names

THE CYNICAL INTERPRETATION

In this interpretation, it should not be surprising that the drug users and their communities were ignored for four or five years; these groups have no political power, and the State Division of Substance Abuse (DSA) is so preoccupied with drug dependency that it sometimes loses sight of the larger goal of saving lives. There is little medical expertise in the agency, and AIDS is not the kind of medical problem that attracts high-quality staff. In any case, until 1984 as many as five times more addicts were dying of overdoses than of AIDS, so initially the DSA's concern was addiction far more than the associated diseases.[36]

In contrast, the gay male population contains a very affluent subcommunity, which had political skills even if the mayor distanced himself and his office from gay groups. Gay men were dying of a new STD but did not want to be treated at the existing STD clinics. Rather, they wanted new programs to deal just with AIDS. One respondent put it this way in an interview: "You simply couldn't ask and expect white gay men, particularly affluent white gay men, to go to sexually transmitted disease clinics that existed at the time, which were currently filled with blacks and Hispanics." Furthermore, they didn't want to call AIDS a sexually transmitted disease because that would ghettoize it; STDs were already an underfunded and stigmatized group of illnesses. An additional problem in using existing STD facilities was that if AIDS is classified as a sexually transmitted disease, it opens up the whole discussion of contact tracing—with whom have you had sex recently? For confidentiality reasons and to encourage people to present themselves for testing, anonymity had to be guaranteed. If AIDS services were located within STD clinics it would be very easy for politicians and clinicians to argue for contact tracing under the provisions that existed for other sexually transmitted diseases. Although this would limit the spread of the disease by warning people about their HIV-positive partners and encouraging them

---

as "muddling through" in political science, "bounded rationality" in psychology, and "garbage can theory" in organizational theory. It is associated with the distinguished names of Charles E. Lindblom, Herbert A. Simon, and James G. March. For a recent exposition, see Perrow, *Complex Organizations*, pp. 119–146.
36. Des Jarlais, Friedman, and Strug, "AIDS and Needle Sharing."

to be tested so that they would not spread the disease inadvertently, there were disadvantages to the approach as well. People would fear to be tested, it was argued, because if the news of a positive result leaked out (a fair possibility) they would lose many of their civil rights. Contact tracing in the case of syphilis has little danger because the disease is tolerated more than AIDS and is not fatal.

The solution was to give the gay community different treatment options —AIDS units in hospitals, with special teams—and to allow the community itself to run whatever education activities would take place.[37] (This meant that the bathhouses would remain open.) The emerging gay group concerned exclusively with AIDS among homosexual men, the Gay Men's Health Crisis, soon held some of the biggest fund-raising events in the city's history. The group would have a say in the handling of the disease and would head up important coordinating committees, but there would be precious little new money from the state or city to go with that say. The rest of the health system, and housing, would stand aside and, when required to act, would set up special devices to keep the disease segregated.

Those who accepted this cynical interpretation of the strategy of centralized fiscal control and segregation of the disease viewed it as positive in only one respect: it had the virtue of forestalling a medical research model of the crisis. New York State Health Commissioner David Axelrod was primarily interested in supporting medical research on the problem; but although research was needed, people were dying, and there was no preventive education. In the cynical view, the federal government should be forced to undertake the medical research; state funds should not be used to build up the New York State research establishment—already the finest state establishment in the nation. In addition, a medical research

37. Actually, the gay community was as confused as everyone else over the issue of separate facilities for AIDS patients. Perhaps the leading AIDS hospital in the country in 1983, San Francisco General, was about to open a special AIDS ward because of the unusual medical demands of these patients. But the head of the Office of Gay and Lesbian Health Concerns argued that AIDS wards would become nothing more than leper colonies. Shilts, *And the Band Played On*, p. 248. Whether to merge or segregate the patients is still a matter of debate. Special units are recommended in the *Report of the Presidential Commission*, p. 17.

model would ignore the issues of discrimination, housing, insurance problems, the need for "buddies," and so on. Giving money to medical research was the safest option for state and city officials playing to an electorate that was overwhelmingly disapproving of people with AIDS and how they got it, and it was feared that the commissioner and the governor were interested only in that. Commissioner Axelrod obliged this interpretation by telling a legislative hearing in 1983, where his inaction was criticized, that hypertension was a more important state health issue in New York.[38]

Leaving the local male gay community to respond to the AIDS crisis meant that the state with all its resources was allowed to take a distancing role, emphasizing coordination rather than direct service when it finally did have to act. (In fact, the city and the state governments formed a series of coordinating groups, the New York State AIDS Institute (1983), the New York City AIDS Consortium (1986), and, in 1988, the New York State AIDS Alert. Two of these, the AI and the AIDS Alert, were headed by gay activists from GMHC.) With the white homosexual community left to raise its own funds and mount its own education campaign, the IVDUs and the gay men and bisexuals in the minority community were virtually ignored. But the deaths kept coming, and the New York City statistics were making headlines across the nation.

CRITICISM OF THE AIDS INSTITUTE

In the cynics' view, the AIDS Institute is a good example of a conduit into the gay male community that provides funds and stems

38. Shilts, p. 340. This was the season when the Republican-dominated State Senate unanimously approved a bill allocating $4.5 million for AIDS research and $700,000 for education and prevention, and Governor Cuomo threatened to veto it, claiming that it was a good bill if the money was available, but the state did not have the money. Later he reversed himself and supported it. See Susan Chira, "Cuomo Says State Will Step Up AIDS Research"; and the section on "AIDS Research" in Edward A. Gargan, "Partisan Dispute Delays Bill to Mitigate Shoreham's Cost." In the next year, 1984, Cuomo failed to put any AIDS money in the budget, so the legislature voted $1.2 million for research and $400,000 for education.

criticism but that keeps the funding small and the strings conservative. When AI teamed up with the New York City AIDS Service Delivery Consortium, which was supported by the national Public Health Service and the Robert Wood Johnson Foundation, the funding for programs increased, but the approach remained cautious. Our interviews brought out a number of specific criticisms.

The AIDS Institute was headed up for years by a gay activist from the Gay Men's Health Crisis, and for this reason it was charged with attempting to buy off the homosexual community. (But, we might note, it was that same community that knew the most about the disease and was doing the most through an unprecedented level of volunteer work and steady fundraising.) The AI was accused by one of our respondents of focusing too heavily on gay males and neglecting women with AIDS and IVDUs. This criticism was openly expressed at meetings called by AI. Others criticized it for spending its resources on coordination when there were so few services to coordinate. Direct funding of services, whether the services were provided by the local groups or the massive city and state health systems, would have been more productive, in this view. (One respondent noted that San Francisco funded service programs while New York State and City funded coordinating bureaucracies.) Still others criticized the AI for funding established programs that were frequently conservative in their health policies and their political views, such as a Brooklyn drug clinic headed by a politically conservative minority leader who supported President Reagan and his view that AIDS education should be restricted to calls for abstinence.

The experience of one activist organization that stirs things up in the city and that receives "establishment" funds throws into relief the conservative official response. The tiny drug-treatment group ADAPT was one of three Brooklyn agencies that applied for funds from the New York State AIDS Consortium, which has close ties to the AIDS Institute. The three groups were told to pool their applications and coordinate their efforts. One of the three, larger than ADAPT, emerged as a dominant member of the trio and now effectively controls the funds. Although ADAPT is a member of the AIDS Consortium, it reportedly has little influence on policy. But is is one of the very few groups with any experience in the minority community and, despite its minuscule size (three staffers and about twenty volunteers in the fall of 1987), it has a national reputation for innovative outreach. (We will discuss it more fully in Chapter 6.) But ADAPT appears to be marginal to the AIDS Institute and to city efforts.

Finally, many said that the AIDS Institute follows the "bureaucracy as usual" model during a crisis that demands unusual risks and flexibility. Applications for grants of $50,000 can run to 100 pages; a small community organization simply cannot manage that. Elaborate workshops are conducted in the World Trade Center in downtown Manhattan to teach small community groups how to apply for funds. The complaint is echoed in a study of two minority communities in New York City by a public health research team. The director of one of the centers that was asked to address the AIDS-prevention issue said, "We need administrative support to be of any assistance. I can't just do a mailing. That takes a lot of work. Our funding is just too tight."[39] Unrealistic ceilings were set on salaries; the maximum salary for the director of a large coordinating and service-giving office was $35,000; that for a smaller organization, $23,000, later changed to $25,000, we were told. Given living costs in New York City and the demands of the jobs, these are pitiful sums.

Except for medical research, there is a serious staffing problem in the AIDS area. The novelty and cross-disciplinary nature of the problem mean that few are qualified, and we suspect that the depressing nature of the disease and perhaps its stigma mean that few of those qualified are willing to make even minor career changes to work on the AIDS problem. Understaffing can perhaps be solved only by paying super-salaries, except where community support through volunteer efforts runs high, as in reasonably well-off parts of San Francisco and Manhattan. We were struck by the dedication (and low salaries) of several of our respondents; the city and the state are lucky to have them. But of course a sound AIDS program cannot depend on finding a few people like these.

39. Freudenberg, Lee, and Silver, "How Minority Community Organizations Respond to the AIDS Epidemic." Many of the findings in this paper are consistent with ours, though our samples and research efforts were completely independent.

Finally, respondents felt that AI did not express an all-out commitment to alleviating the epidemic in the black and Hispanic communities. It was a matter of luck that the Brooklyn community program, which was making a difference through an exceptional administrator, gave the AI a foothold in that borough, but the institute had little going elsewhere. The Harlem initiative, just starting in 1988 was four years late; efforts in the drug-using community were equally late. The view of respondents in New York City, then, contrasted sharply with the evaluation by George Washington University researchers in their comprehensive study for the Public Health Service, which described the institute as "innovative" and "imaginative."[40]

THE INSTITUTE'S VIEW

The response of the AIDS Institute staff was as follows. The state, including the governor and the health commissioner, had a full commitment to AIDS. When asked why the state was so slow to fund programs, the uniform reply was that initially everyone had failed to realize how serious the crisis would become. (The California record, the pleas from the Gay Men's Health Crisis and other groups, the warnings from CDC experts, and even the appropriations of the state legislature, over the threat of a veto by the governor, would seem to contradict this excuse.) The supposed segregation of AIDS was vigorously denied, and with good arguments. The staff would not comment on the strategy of Mayor Koch. In fact, they noted that relationships with the city administration per se left much to be desired, and there was admittedly no joint long-range planning. The lack of a joint planning mechanism was a remarkable omission, one would think, for a state health institute located in the city where the vast majority of cases were found. ("I don't know what the City is doing," said the head of the New York City office in disgust.) But the governor and legislature had created the institute for good reason: the effort should not be in the governor's office because he should not have to bear "the political fallout." It should be within the Public Health

40. Intergovernmental Health Policy Project, *Assessing the Problem*, p. 1–17.

Department because there was no other sensible place to put it; after all, AIDS was a health matter. But by creating an institute, instead of parcelling out the tasks among the infectious disease, drug abuse, housing, and social service units, supporters said, the administration would gain expertise, focus, and the all-important ability to contract out and thus move more quickly. Even the matter of civil service approval for new staff positions and community workers could slow things up if the existing bureaucracies tried to add them.

As cogent as this argument is, it is still the case that the AI was formed late, was given little money, and moved slowly and cautiously in contracting out. Of course the AIDS Institute had to give contracts to the GMHC; it would have been accused of massive homophobia if it ignored the gay men, especially since they were literally providing the only services in town three years into the crisis. Its other contracts in the first year went to conventional organizations that provided few services, and almost none went to the minority community. (A hospital did some educational outreach; the Red Cross provided transportation; and so on.)

THE MINORITY COMMUNITY AND AIDS

As feeble as services are for the gay male community, they appear to be even less vigorous for black and Hispanic gay men, IVDUs in the ghettoes, and the impoverished white IVDUs, except in the extreme case of emergency room admissions. Perhaps as many as 2,500 active AIDS cases in late 1988 were unaccounted for by the legitimate agencies —hospitals, hospices, AIDS housing, and what we know of those PWAs with the resources to receive care in their homes.

Two possibilities exist to explain why such a large population receives care only in extremity: the funds are not available for health care and community services, in which case the AI is quite wrong about the funding levels of the state government (and city officials are wrong about the city's funding response); or there is no place to send funds, in which case state and city officials are correct because they have sent all the funds that could be absorbed. In our view both possibilities are true: there were very few funds available, but there were limited places to

send those that were made available. More money could well have generated organizations capable of using it, but that did not happen during
the 1980s.

The organizational failure of the AIDS Institute is tied in part only,
but still in significant part, to the organizational poverty of the minority
communities. That in turn is due to the deterioration of these communities since the early 1970s. A negative synergetic effect between AIDS
and the problems of extreme poverty has made the impact of AIDS on
the black and Hispanic populations more severe than could be expected
from other types of deadly epidemics. In order to understand this effect,
we must pause to examine the minority communities, black and Hispanic,
in New York City.

6   MINORITIES AND AIDS IN

NEW YORK CITY

Historic discrimination against blacks and Hispanics underlies the current problems of the poorest of the poor, the underclass. The booming economy of the World War II years brought more prosperity to the black community than it had ever had, and that carried over into the 1950s and the 1960s, but since then, to continuing racial discrimination, reduced only somewhat by the protests and legislation of the 1960s, has been added profound "structural" changes in the economy that eroded many gains Americans of color had made. William Wilson, in *The Truly Disadvantaged*, provides a convincing account of these changes and the problems that followed. The manufacturing jobs that black migrants, pushed out of the South by the technological revolution in agriculture there, had once taken in the North began to be replaced by service jobs. Most of the 8 million new jobs created in the Reagan years were low-skilled service jobs, but they were disproportionately in the suburbs and not in the central city, where the blacks and increasingly the Hispanic migrants were. The central city needed fairly skilled service jobs, from secretaries and filing clerks on up to stockbrokers. This was especially true of New York City, which saw manufacturing sharply decline and finance and real estate boom. For instance, between 1970 and 1984 there was a decrease of 34 percent in New York City's jobs requiring less than a high school education; over the same period, the number of jobs requiring some college increased by

24 percent.[1] (This trend is continuing and intensifying.)[2] The result is that unemployment among minorities is more than twice as high as unemployment among mainstream whites.

Structural economic changes occurred while a major real estate boom was taking place in the city, a boom fueled by the large tax advantages offered by the Koch administration,[3] as the whole Northeast prospered largely because of the massive increase in defense spending. The "gentrification" of neighborhoods pushed the poor out, at the same time the number of poor increased through high birth rates and, for a time, continuing in-migration. Spending by the federal government on housing declined sharply in this period, and the state and city did not take up the slack. The result was homelessness, particularly among the minorities, who saw first their jobs, then affordable housing disappear.

Joblessness and homelessness have raised family-dissolution indicators to levels twice as high as twenty or thirty years ago. For example, between 1959 and the mid-1980s the percent of poor black families headed by women went from 30 to 74, and the percent of all births that took place out of wedlock went from 24 to 57 percent. Wilson attributes much of this staggering phenomenon to the "shrinking marriageable pool" of economically stable black males. Female-headed families are overwhelmingly poor, whether white or black. They earn just 43 percent of the mean income of husband-wife families; if the female is black, they earn only 37 percent of husband-wife families.[4] Poverty and homelessness are the sequels of widespread joblessness and family dislocation of the minority communities living in the inner city.

In addition, the black and Hispanic communities are on the average younger than the mainstream community. Poorly educated young persons are more likely to be out of the labor force, to get involved in crime, and to become drug addicts. These demographic factors inter-

1. Wilson, *The Truly Disadvantaged*, p. 40.
2. Figures for other cities—such as Baltimore, Boston, St. Louis, and Philadelphia —look even worse in relative terms, although New York City's population size makes the problem much more worrisome there than anywhere else.
3. Newfield and Barrett, *City for Sale*.
4. Wilson, p. 27.

act with the economic changes to the further disadvantage of poor communities.

Social dislocation leads to other problems. First, phenomena such as crime, drug addiction, poor schooling, and higher school dropout rates flow from and add to the problems of poverty and homelessness. Second, social dislocation at the individual and family levels leads to the social isolation of the minority community. The problems become less visible to the affluent parts of the city; the social programs find it harder to penetrate and work in the ghettos; the reasonably successful minority members flee the inner city and leave the less well off without the role models of people who go to work every day and learn the ways of the dominant classes; grass-roots groups do not have successful professionals and business people to draw upon for leadership and small funds; languages and dialects become more private and isolated. And social isolation excludes people from the job networks that permeate more prosperous neighborhoods.[5]

In brief, a large number of black and Hispanic children are born into long-term poverty and, the chances are great, into welfare-dependent families. Welfare dependency does not increase social dislocation per se, as some studies by conservative writers suggest, but it does augment social isolation from the job networks and, in general, from mainstream society.[6] Those who have stayed in the depressed inner cities are said to form an underclass rather than merely a poor lower class. The white poor outnumber the nonwhite poor, but they are not concentrated in impoverished communities with barely no ties with mainstream society.

Blacks and other minorities come, in a sense, at the tail end of a major social upheaval, and they are whiplashed by the force of change to a greater degree than the majority community. For example, drug use has been declining significantly in the majority community. The 1988 National Household Survey on Drug Abuse found a 37 percent decline from a 1985 survey in the number of people who said they had used

---

5. Wilson, p. 57; and Massey and Denton, "Hypersegregation in U.S. Metropolitan Areas."
6. This particular point is well argued in Wilson, pp. 16–18.

marijuana, cocaine, and other illicit drugs in the previous month. Over the three years, there was a 25 percent drop in the number who said they had ever used an illegal drug. These are striking changes, especially since the supply of drugs is plentiful and their price has declined.

But at the same time the total number of heavy cocaine users, including those using crack, rose sharply from 1985 to 1988, by 33 percent for those using it once a week or more and by 19 percent for daily and almost-daily users. Although casual use of cocaine had dropped more than the use of other illicit drugs in the general population (by 50 percent), the proportion of black and Hispanic people using it had not changed. Thus, the minority communities are the last to experience a drop in drug use, and any drop in casual use there is offset by the sharp rise in the number of heavy users of cocaine.[7]

A similar phenomenon occurs with hepatitis B, an inflammation of the liver caused by a virus that can be spread through blood, semen, and vaginal fluids. While it is treatable, it can be deadly and in 6–10 percent of the cases it leads to chronic liver disease and associated deaths. A vaccine has been available for some years, but in the past decade the number of cases has increased to 300,000 per year, from 200,000 earlier. The rise is primarily in the minority community. The percentage of cases among homosexuals has dropped sharply as they have modified their sexual behavior, and they are now only the third-largest risk group. Heterosexuals with multiple partners constitute the second-largest risk group, and intravenous drug users the largest risk group—again, the minority community.[8] Syphilis has been declining for decades, but it is sharply up in the minority community—up 50 percent.[9] Homicide, too, is on the rise in minority communities. In St. Louis, the Missouri State Department of Health reported that at this rate, "1 out of every 13 black males in St. Louis who is 15 years old will be murdered by the time he is 45."[10] (Such figures, along with the numbers of tuberculosis and

7. "Casual Drug Use Is Sharply Down."
8. Altman, "As Hepatitis B Spreads, Physicians Reconsider Vaccination Strategy."
9. Mahar, "Pitiless Scourge," p. 16.
10. "Black Men in St. Louis Slain at Highest Rate."

AIDS cases, help give substance to the charge of racial genocide by minority community leaders.) Tuberculosis has been declining since the early part of this century, except, in the past decade, in large cities and particularly in the poor minority parts of those cities. It is fueled by homelessness, poor diet, and stress, and now it interacts with AIDS.

ENTER AIDS

One result of the increasing polarization between the majority and minority populations, the white and the nonwhite, has been that poverty and discrimination are apparently escalating afflictions that are being removed from the majority population. To the extents that AIDS can be parsed in these terms it too is declining, not in absolute numbers, but in the rate of infection, among whites (primarily gay men), but the rate of infection is rising among minorities (gay men, IVDUs, and their sexual partners and offspring).

AIDS does not merely add to the burdens of the inner-city poor in cities such as New York; it is not a case of adding one unit of disaster to four existing units to get five. AIDS has helped to increase the size of existing units by intensifying their impact and increasing their resistance to change. To take a simple example, the housing shortage that has led to homelessness also produces conditions that spread AIDS (by putting people with HIV into situations where sex and cheap drugs are more readily exchanged), causing neighborhoods to deteriorate and thus further decreasing the stock of usable housing, leading to more homelessness, which spreads the virus. Homeless shelters are becoming major centers for the spread of the virus. A recent study found a 62 percent infection rate among shelter dwellers.[11]

AIDS comes to a minority community whose members, in comparison with mainstream whites, are disproportionately young, jobless, homeless, poorly educated, and addicted to IV drugs. Thus, high-risk behaviors such as unstable, multiple sexual partnerships and needle-sharing are more common than in mainstream communities. Homelessness and

---

11. Lambert, "Study Finds Alarming AIDS Rate in Homeless Shelter."

poor education are major obstacles to the dissemination of information about how to prevent infection. First, the homeless are a group difficult to target with conventional mass-media education programs; they are simply more difficult to locate. Second, poorly educated people are less likely to pay attention to explanations about the ways in which one can get infected. Education is already playing a major role in preventing further spread of the disease among gay white men, according to recent government reports.[12] But minority groups are not being buffered from the disease with preventive education to the extent that mainstream groups have been. A dramatic case is that of IVDUs, most of whom lack stable jobs, family ties, or homes.

Community-based or grass-roots organization has been a major resource for coping with AIDS for other affected groups, such as white, middle-class gays. Grass-roots organizations have been very successful in conducting preventive and health care programs. Yet, minority communities face pathetic prospects for large-scale self-organization owing to their dislocation, impoverishment, and isolation from mainstream society. Neither fundraising nor volunteering is easy when communities have to deal with the problems of joblessness, homelessness, crime, drug addiction, discrimination, and family dissolution. The larger picture is one of overburdened agendas and also of multiplicative factors. For example, population-targeted, culture-specific AIDS education becomes more important with people who are homeless or jobless. It is also widely accepted that the organizational tool most likely to succeed in outreach programs is a grass-roots group. Yet those two demands happen to be contradictory in the case of minority IVDUs: they need targeted education but have few prospects for self-organization.[13]

Minority people are not only more likely to engage in high-risk behavior and less likely to have help from community groups; they are also

12. Office of Technology Assessment, *How Effective Is AIDS Education?* See also the study for the National Research Council reported in Turner, Miller, and Moses, eds., *AIDS*, pp. 259–356; and Institute of Medicine, *Confronting AIDS: Update 1988* (Washington, D.C.: National Academy Press, 1988), pp. 64–69.

13. For a discussion, see Samuel R. Friedman and Cathy Casriel, "Drug Users' Organizations and AIDS Policy."

less likely to get appropriate health care once the immune deficiency brings about its inescapable consequences. If employed, blacks and Hispanics are less likely to have generous health care benefits than are mainstream people in mainstream jobs. If they are welfare-dependent but homeless, they will find that hospitals have an incentive not to diagnose them as having AIDS in that federal regulations ban hospitals from discharging homeless patients. If they are jobless and lack welfare protection, they will find it difficult to get adequate health care at a time when hospitals are overcrowded, primary care and nursing is scarce, and health care financing is in trouble. Minorities die several months sooner, on average, after an AIDS diagnosis than do whites, but it is not their genetic character that makes the difference. It is that they are in poorer health and delay longer in seeking treatment because of the lack of facilities and the social barriers.[14]

Under these conditions, it is not surprising that the biggest increase in AIDS in recent years has been among minorities. In the Unites States, white males still constitute the majority of AIDS cases (56 percent), living and dead, but in New York City the minorities already account for the majority of the cases (60 percent). What is more important, blacks and Hispanics represent 64 percent of the cases reported in the twelve months before August 1989.[15]

In the United States as a whole there are fourteen times as many black women and nine times as many Hispanic women with AIDS than white women, and the rates for black and Hispanic children are fifteen and nine times higher, respectively, than for white children. Overall, 40 percent of American AIDS cases are black or Hispanic, though these groups are only about 20 percent of the population.[16]

14. Mays Cochran, "Acquired Immunodeficiency Syndrome and Black Americans."

15. Data for the United States calculated by the difference between the cumulative reported cases between 2 April 15, 1988, and November 19, 1989; Centers for Disease Control, *HIV / AIDS Surveillance Report*, p. 9. Data for New York City supplied by the AIDS Surveillance Unit, New York City Department of Health. See also AIDS Surveillance Unit, *AIDS Surveillance Update*, pp. 6 and 10.

16. The best sources for statistics are the following: Carbine and Lee, *AIDS into the 90's*; Fineberg, "The Social Dimensions of AIDS"; Friedman et al., "The

There are two major differences between the white and minority communities with respect to AIDS among adults. First, among whites, 80 percent of the cases are gay or bisexual non-IVDUs, whereas in the minority community the figure is 40 percent. Note that sexual orientation still plays a large role—40 percent—in the minority community. Second, only 12 percent of white males with AIDS are IVDUs (or the sex partners of women who used IV drugs), but 40 percent of the black and Hispanic men with AIDS fall into that category. Drug use or involvement with a male user is associated with 48 percent of white women with AIDS, 70 percent of black women, and 83 percent of Hispanic women. In large cities in the Northeast, IVDUs are the majority of new AIDS cases, with infection rates estimated at 50 percent or more, and over 80 percent of these are minorities. Blacks and Hispanics constitute over half of the AIDS cases in New York, Philadelphia, Baltimore, Newark, Miami, and Washington, D.C. On the West Coast, the infection rate among IVDUs is still very low, around 5 percent, and the proportion of minorities among AIDS cases is much lower than in the East.

Thus, it is in the minority communities of the East Coast that AIDS is striking the hardest, and it is affecting women and children to an alarming degree. A hospital in Newark that serves primarily poor blacks and Hispanics reported in 1988 that one out of every twenty-three babies was born to a mother infected with the AIDS virus; half of these newborns are infected themselves and have a high chance of developing the disease early in childhood.[17] AIDS has become a disease of the family in these environments, with father, mother, and child infected, and just one more problem, even if the last, for these families. The infant mortality rate in the ghettos was already three times the rate in white areas, and higher than the infant mortality rate of forty of the "underdeveloped"

AIDS Epidemic among Blacks and Hispanics"; and Krieger, *The Politics of AIDS*. We appreciate the excellent undergraduate seminar paper by Amy M. Robohm, who pulled together much of this material. See also the more recent *AIDS Information Sourcebook, 1988–1989*, edited by H. Robert Malinowsky and Gerald J. Perry.

17. Williams, "Inner City under Siege."

nations of the world.[18] There is not much of a health system ready to inform these families about AIDS, let alone allow them to die in some dignity. Isolation, poverty, homelessness, and lack of health care have been magnified by AIDS.

CULTURE, RELIGION, AND POLITICS

Thus far we have argued that AIDS has multiplied or exacerbated the conditions underlying the minority community's dislocation and isolation from mainstream society. Increased risk of infection, more difficult grass-roots organization, and less access to health care have resulted from the interaction of AIDS with already existing social dislocation and isolation. The problem of AIDS in the minority communities becomes even more complicated when culture, religion, and politics are taken into account.

Consider cultural factors first. Using a condom and cleaning IV "works" are quite simple acts, and even taking these precautions half the time would have a significant effect on the propagation of the virus. But patterns of male dominance and indifference to risks—that is, "macho" behavior—in minority communities appear to be strong. In our interviews we repeatedly heard that black and Hispanic homosexuals and bisexuals hid their sexual orientation from their female sex partners. We also were told that young black males and especially young Hispanic males engaged in homosexual acts without thinking of themselves as homosexual or bisexual. These cultural characteristics, adaptive in themselves, no doubt, encouraged the spread of AIDS.[19]

Newspaper reports supported our interview material. Lena Williams, writing in the *New York Times*, notes: "Many black and Hispanic men, for example, refuse to use condoms, viewing them as something for homosexuals. And even when the men are intravenous drug users, their wives or lovers are afraid to ask them to use condoms." Women in these cultures may be especially vulnerable to demands for anal sex and

18. Green, "End the Cutbacks."
19. See Turner, Miller, and Moses, eds., *AIDS*, p. 119, for ethnographic evidence of the "macho" behavior in IVDU couples.

condom-free sex because their poverty makes the male's threat of walking out on them, if he is providing support, potent.[20]

The culture of the inner city is also a very suspicious one. The residents reportedly are suspicious of governmental attempts to help them. Those whose immigrant status is not very secure fear that they may be deported and are not likely to seek AIDS testing. Furthermore, if knowledge of their positive status were to be available in the community, they fear isolation and scorn. At present, AIDS appears to be far less accepted as a fact of life that must be dealt with in a humane, nonjudgmental way in the minority community than in the white community—where this degree of acceptance is already woefully low.

One of the most powerful integrative forces in the minority communities is the church. Indeed, the church is *the* organization of note in these communities. Without the support of the Catholic Church in the Hispanic communities and the Protestant churches in the black communities, no extensive educational program can proceed, housing for AIDS patients will be difficult to provide, new drug clinics will be denied suitable space, and even shelters for the homeless will not be made available. It is a tragic irony of the AIDS epidemic in the minority communities that the one organizational force that could be mobilized to fight the disease has refused to acknowledge the problem for years and has resisted attempts to enlist its aid, though there are signs that this is beginning to change.

The Catholic Church is well known for its adamant resistance to AIDS education that includes references to condoms. It shares this repulsion of safe nonmarital sex with many black church leaders, perhaps most of them. To show an example of the logic and feeling of some black church leaders, we will draw upon a striking documentary aired by National Public Radio's program "All Things Considered" in April 1989. The interviews and commentary were by Brenda Wilson, who recorded speeches at a meeting of black ministers in Philadelphia earlier that year. The meeting was called to bring leading ministers together to discuss the position their churches should take on the AIDS crisis in their

20. Williams, "Inner City under Siege."

communities. As an indication of the problem, the meeting took three years to set up; 400 were invited, 150 came. It appears that those opposed to any action other than condemning the "sinful behavior" that leads to AIDS were in the majority.

The ministers grappled with a difficult issue: the best protection against AIDS is education, but education in this case would instruct the "students" how to "sin" without getting infected. A church whose mission in the past had been not only to save souls but to hide slaves, educate newly freed persons, initiate the civil rights movement and support it through its violent history, and then as now to house, feed, and clothe poor black people was being asked to go into crack houses and shooting galleries and give out condoms and bleach kits.

Said the Reverend David Weeks of Shalom Baptist Church in his minisermon on the theology of AIDS:

> For the theology of AIDS, I hear Jesus saying it is better for man to go into life all maimed and blind than have all his members cast into hell's fire.
>
> I dare say, on the theology of AIDS, those folks who know they are going to die may get right with God more than those folks who we are dealing with who *don't know* they are going to die.
>
> So on the theology of AIDS, when you get to heaven you might find *more* AIDS victims *up there*.
>
> You understand what I am saying? Get some of those other folks you been dealing with.
>
> So you can't come up and tell me clearly, here is the position of the church; the church has got to work that out.
>
> We got to show love, compassion, and care, and yet not get ourselves caught up with *aiding and abetting* doing things that God *clearly condemns*.

Brenda Wilson comments that by this time one of the leaders of the group, a Howard University professor of divinity, the Reverend Dr. Calvin Morris, had taken his suit coat off and loosened his tie. "Somewhat gingerly," she continues, "as if to defuse the tension, [Dr. Morris] responded that he would hate to think that you would have to kill off half the black community to make sure they get into heaven." But for the ministers, extramarital sex is fornication, homosexuality is an abomination, drug abuse is a crime against the laws of God and man, and people with AIDS contract it through sin. "God is not going to change his position on sin," one minister proclaimed. But Morris persisted.

> My brothers and sisters, I have heard ministers say that, because of the activities and proclivities of gay people and drug abusers, what is happening to them is God's judgment. We have to struggle with that kind of theology because we know if that was the case, if sinful folk got their just deserts, most white folk would have been dead a long time ago. If God dealt with us according to our sins where would we be?

But for at least some it was, in Wilson's words, "far better that a person die even from AIDS with his soul ready to meet God." The person who could sin with impunity, using the condoms and bleach kits provided by activist ministers, would not be prepared.

In New York City, as in much of the nation, this cultural position, shared with the Catholic archdiocese and so consistent with the "moral majority," is echoed in part by many who represent the other important force in the minority community, their political leaders. Black and Hispanic political representatives have not been in the forefront of education campaigns, or even very explicit about the AIDS threat, though that may be changing slowly. In June 1989, some eight years into the epidemic, ten of New York City's leading black clergymen broke what they said was the silence of many blacks about AIDS. They sought to mobilize nearly 600 black congregations in the area by the next fall. Some churches had even refused to hold burials for people who had died of AIDS. Though strongly opposed to the distribution of free needles, the Reverend Calvin O. Butts III of the Abyssinian Baptist Church in Harlem declared, "People are becoming more enlightened and realize it's a problem we have to combat."[21] Black politicians in New York City have been vociferous in their opposition to the distribution of free nee-

21. Lambert, "Black Clergy Set to Preach about AIDS."

dles and to the establishment of "no-frill" methadone clinics, a subject
we shall explore in Chapter 7. To give just one example here, New York
City Councilman Hilton B. Clark of Harlem "recently accused the
New York City Health Commissioner, Dr. Stephen C. Joseph, of using
the free needle program to conduct a *genocidal* campaign against black
and Hispanic people." To which Yolanda Serrano, executive director of ADAPT, said, "Where were they for the last eight years? It's
genocide now while blacks and Latinos are dying in the streets from
AIDS."[22]

"THE BEST POSSIBLE RESPONSE"?

We believe that the efforts of New York State and City, and of
the AIDS Institute in particular, have been late, feeble, and totally incom-
mensurate with the scope of the challenge. But, as our brief journey into
the minority community suggests, even if the state, the city, and the
institute had made the appropriate effort, they would have faced enormous hurdles to effective action. It would appear that a multitude of
problems converges on the matter of AIDS education and prevention,
not to speak of simple care, which we have not explored, that makes any
normal organizational response ridiculously inadequate.

The main resistance to outreach in these communities is probably not
to be found in city and state bureaucracies. Virtually everyone we interviewed, including minority respondents working in AIDS programs,
agreed that it was very difficult for the black and Hispanic communities
to deal with AIDS, and for excellent reasons. AIDS was just one more
burden on top of so many others (drugs, crack, poor schools, very poor
health services, unemployment, low skills, lack of housing, rising tuberculosis and syphilis rates, and, above all, rampant crime). So many
people were victims of conditions beyond their control that sympathy for
the victims of drugs and AIDS was in relatively short supply. The stig-

22. Marriott, "Needle Exchange Angers Many Minorities" (emphasis added). See
also Marriott, "New York Alters Needle Plan to Combat AIDS." The needle plan
was also opposed by Charles Rangel, a liberal black congressman from New York.

matized minority community could stigmatize their IVDUs and gay men and bisexuals quite easily; they knew about stigmas.

We think, therefore, that there are three reasons for the poor organizational response in the minority community: (1) most organizations in the community were unwilling to face the AIDS problem and did not apply for or press for funds; (2) the community has few appropriate organizations in its midst to receive the funds; (3) it does not have an infrastructure that is capable of absorbing the funds (where there are organizations, they do not have the trained personnel for the new tasks or a supportive political structure; they have a culture that makes access to families difficult for outsiders; and there are even simple problems such as safe transportation for the ill, families, and health workers).

AIDS Institute staffers, not surprisingly, tended to say that the problem was more with the minority community and with the delayed realization that AIDS was not strictly a "gay disease" than with the state or the AIDS Institute itself. There *is* evidence that part of the problem lies within the minority community. It was hard to get communities to submit proposals; some boroughs with many AIDS cases had never submitted them, others had to be coaxed, and the institute had to play an active role in drafting acceptable proposals. So even if the organizational infrastructure existed, the relevant organizations were unresponsive. Part of the problem might lie in the sheer technical demands of proposal writing, and we heard complaints on that score; it would indicate that the infrastructure, if it existed, was geared to direct community needs rather than the more bureaucratic expectations of the state. Meetings in the World Trade Center to explain the complex proposals are not appropriate. (The institute proudly pointed out that the most recent round of requests was kicked off with an initial meeting of community groups, city agencies, and the institute held in Harlem. The change in location would seem to be a mild inconvenience for the state agency.)

The organizing force for the minority community was the church, and it was particularly conservative on the issues of drug abuse and what it regarded as sexual deviancy. Community leaders called for forced sterilization of women with AIDS, for example (one of these headed a major AIDS program!), but said little or nothing about caring for them or their children. One of our respondents, a social worker in the AIDS unit of a hospital, made it clear that when she occasionally did outreach work in the black churches in her community she never mentioned safe sex, only abstinence. Media coverage of the heroic work of another respondent (a white, upper-class woman physician working in a hospital that was wretchedly equipped and maintained, according to our interviewer) brought a small response for volunteers to help with pediatric AIDS cases, but they were all white and soon left. The time budget and resources of the poor are not adequate for the kind of volunteer work that could take place in Manhattan's gay community or in the white community, and the stigma attached to AIDS in the black community probably exceeds that in the majority community.

The problem is vastly more difficult to cope with in minority communities where the victims are drug abusers, their female partners, and their children, and the gay and bisexual men who must hide their sexual orientation far more than in the majority community; all are to some degree underground in a community that is partly underground anyway.[23] Addressing the problem here is vastly different from working in the gay community, which, although it has its poor whites, is comparatively open about its orientation, affluent, interconnected, politically skilled, and within reach of substantial resources.

In brief, AIDS, more than any other social problem facing the minority community, attacks on two fronts. It attacks the source of social cohesion, religion, by requiring that churches violate their norms and conventions, which are more conservative than even those of the Catholic Church in the white areas. Second, it requires that the posture of masculinity, male dominance, or "macho" behavior, so much a part of the community's defense of its embattled and disintegrating position, be modified or abandoned. Otherwise it will be very difficult to reach homosexual and bisexual males, because they must hide and remain unacknowledged. And it will be difficult for the female partners of male

23. Note that 53 percent of all black men with AIDS and 54 percent of all Hispanic men with AIDS are gay or bisexual. Centers for Disease Control, *HIV / AIDS Surveillance*, p. 10.

IVDUs to insist upon safe sex or to escape from the relationship altogether. Normally, plagues do not strike so cruelly at the few defenses —church and ideology—that an impoverished community has. Furthermore, under the new immigration bill, the consequence of AIDS for many Hispanics is deportation. The leader of a group serving recent immigrants predicted that other Hispanics would be blamed as the Haitians had when they were found to harbor the disease in great numbers. As researchers into this problem point out, "If a group believes that the consequence of calling attention to a problem is going to be further discrimination, it is unlikely to raise the issue."[24]

But the distinctive impact of AIDS upon minorities is only part of the story. Have the city and state governments tried to create and fund education and care programs in the minority community? Not to any great extent, most of our respondents and the record suggest, despite the efforts of the AIDS Institute. (Recall that the city and the state barely did anything for the more vocal and politically powerful gay community; in particular, they failed completely to mount an aggressive education campaign when it could have made a great difference.) By the end of 1985, the problem of AIDS in minority communities was already well established. Fully 34 percent of adult AIDS cases were among IVDUs; black and Hispanic patients accounted for 52 percent of the adult cases. The AIDS Institute had yet to make a serious effort to fund local community groups; its major funding—only $765,000 in 1986—still went to the GMHC, which, fortunately, was beginning to expand its efforts into the minority and IVDU communities.[25] In 1988 we asked a member of the Brooklyn Aids Task Force, the flagship example of AI effort, whether the task force had enough money to carry out the necessary programs. The answer was "certainly not," and a *doubling* of the budget was considered a minimum. The agency indicated that it served only 200 AIDS cases out of 2,500 in the borough, and that at least 60 percent never get help from any agency!

24. Freudenberg, Lee, and Silver, "How Minority Community Organizations Respond to the AIDS Epidemic" (there are no page numbers in this article).
25. Dunne, "New York City," p. 158.

The city's response was even weaker. Health Commissioner Stephen Joseph was the most responsive and concerned, but he inherited a fragmented, cosmetic program, a legacy from the days of the Office of Gay and Lesbian Health Concerns. Poverty and crime appear to be dragging the city under while it focuses on real estate and finance—the two things that determine the power in the city, we were told even by city officials. We interviewed many dedicated and hard-working city employees in the mayor's office, the city council, the Health and Hospitals Corporation, and so on, but they were largely overwhelmed by the AIDS problem. Some resolutely insisted that the city had done everything it could have done but lacked the information that would have prepared it for the problem (one of the major myths of the epidemic) and the resources to handle it. It is true that the fiscal crisis of the late 1970s followed by large cuts in federal programs, such as housing, left the city reeling; New York was unable to expend funds until the prosperity of the mid 1980s. But the initial level of funding that could have made a difference probably would have amounted to only a few real estate tax-relief programs to midtown developers. Meanwhile the minority population, homelessness, unemployment, and associated social problems increased even as speculation drove part of the city to new heights of affluence. AIDS struck a city that was singularly indifferent to and unable to cope with social disaster, a city that gave top priority to growth, the character of its leadership, and the depth of its recently revealed corruption.

7 AIDS AND ORGANIZATIONS:

THE NEW ENTRIES

We have argued and documented that there was a massive organizational failure in the response of existing organizations to the AIDS crisis. Furthermore, we argued that this went beyond "normal" organizational failure and was only partly due to economic and ideological factors. It appeared, when we examined the particular character of the AIDS epidemic, that the failure was due largely to the unique characteristics of AIDS—the stigma of association with male homosexual practices, with illegal drug use, and increasingly with poor minority groups; the fatal nature of the disease and uncertainty about transmission; and the enormous costs that were projected, which threatened to sink organizations and political systems. We saw how these themes played out in New York State and City—in particular, the response of the AIDS Institute, the primary resource for fighting the epidemic, and the problems it faced in working within the minority community. We saw that the minority community, overflowing with tragedy, not only was finding it difficult to cope but was finding that its major institution, the church, was making matters worse, as was its defensive culture of "machoism."

Now we will examine more carefully what individual organizations did. Not only will this history reinforce the thesis that AIDS has been unique, but it will also serve another purpose: it should increase our understanding of organizations in general or, in technical terms, contribute to theories of organizations. We wish to examine the idea that organizations consist in considerable part of defenses against misuse by people from within and without. We will see the advantage of regarding organizations as bundles of defenses against goal distortion, discrimination, and difficult and unpleasant tasks. AIDS, we will argue, overwhelms these defenses more than most challenges have; it leaves organizations vulnerable to what might be called "opportunistic infections."

If the organizations in place largely failed to cope with the new disease, what about the new ones that were formed? Three of these will be considered in the next section: the Gay Men's Health Crisis (GMHC) in New York City, the Shanti Project in San Francisco, and the Association for Drug Abuse Prevention and Treatment (ADAPT) in New York City. These are all successful, but are vastly different in many respects.

THE GAY MEN'S HEALTH CRISIS

The Gay Men's Health Crisis was founded in New York City in January 1982 by a group of gay activists who knew that their health needs were not being met by existing health-care providers. Many of their friends and lovers were coming down with a rare disease that the medical establishment could not explain or treat. This was happening before the disease was known as AIDS. The group decided that some type of organization was needed to respond to the disease in terms of both prevention and care. The men had collected approximately $6,000 to start GMHC. None of the founders held a high position in state or local government agencies; all were well-educated professionals or artists working in a large city that paid little attention to gay activities and concerns.

GMHC grew rapidly during its first months. It was the first and only organization, public, private, or voluntary, to provide education, prevention, and counseling services to the gay male population in the city. By October 1982, barely ten months after its birth, GMHC had a volunteer force of over three hundred individuals and was training up to fifty new volunteers every month. At this time, the organization "was running its entire operation out of five small rooms in a boarding house," because neither private landlords nor the city wanted to provide the site for New

York's "leper central."[1] In addition to logistical concerns the fledgling organization had to contend with uncertainties about a new disease of which little was known.[2] For example, meetings would focus on what volunteers should be taught to do, what kinds of services PWAs needed, and how to raise money for services.

During its first two years of existence, GMHC's funds came largely from individual contributions. In 1983, the organization discovered that special benefit events like the famous Madison Square Garden circus could significantly increase revenues, and it has continued to sponsor fundraisers. Over time the source of contributions has depended less on affluent gay men and more on foundations and institutions. But the critical change in GMHC's finances occurred when state and local government began funding the organization, an event with implications for GMHC's internal power structure and educational policies.

Government grants and contracts from New York State began playing a substantial role in the GMHC after mid-1983, accounting for up to one-third of the organization's budget as early as 1984. This was the time when the state founded the AIDS Institute, a coordinating body presided over by a former officer of GMHC. It was also the moment when the board of directors of the GMHC split over the issues of whether gay men should be told to stop having sex altogether and whether bathhouses should be shut down.[3] Initially playwright Larry Kramer (*The Normal Heart*), one of the founders and an energetic grass-roots activist, took the radical stand of proposing that gays should be advised not to have sex at all, presumably because even condoms might not be sufficient protection. GMHC president and Wall Street businessman Paul Popham and his successor, Richard Dunne, argued that gay men should be provided with neutral information and should decide for themselves whether to have safe sex or to risk their lives practicing unprotected sex; that is, they proposed an "informed choice" strategy. But they never thought that abstinence from all kinds of sexual activity was a necessary step to prevent the spread of the virus.

1. Shilts, *And the Band Played On*, p. 380.
2. Shilts, pp. 166–167.
3. Shilts, p. 210.

Popham and Kramer also diverged on what the focus of GMHC's activities should be. Popham wanted GMHC to create a network of social services for gay men while Kramer preferred to concentrate on making the city government organize the required services.[4] The internal struggle eventually ended when Kramer was expelled from the board of directors. (He later tried to reenter but his requests were defeated.)[5] GMHC, originally a fairly innovative organization, was learning the ropes and would avoid political confrontations. Just eighteen months after its birth, at the U.S. Conference of Mayors in June 1983, GMHC impressed the participants with carefully presented documentation, including flowcharts and formal job descriptions, that "to President Popham were the stuff of a sound organization."[6] An organizational chart presented to one of our interviewers in late 1987 included over eighty formal positions or offices arranged into seven distinct directorships: public information, finance and administration, client services, education, legal services, media information program, and development.

The key officials of the GMHC—stockbrokers, publishers, directors, doctors, and the like—presumably knew how to run a sound organization. This is not a trivial matter, as will be evident in the sections on ADAPT and the Shanti Project, below. The organizational ability of GMHC probably reflects the gay culture of New York City, in contrast to, say, that of San Francisco, the only other city with a large homosexual population. Gay men in New York City were still "in the closet," it was widely believed, compared with the openness of San Francisco's gays, and perhaps they were more likely to be in respectable professions. Larry Kramer, frozen out of the bureaucratic structure, had to start his own organization, the Aids Coalition to Unleash Power, or ACT UP, and deliberately kept the bureaucratic apparatus to a minimum. A small but sharp gadfly, ACT UP had significant success in 1989 and 1990 in speeding up trials for new drugs and calling attention to pharmaceutical companies' prices and profits.

If we keep in mind a "straight" world gradually and reluctantly real-

4. Shilts, pp. 166–167.
5. Shilts, pp. 418 and 484.
6. Shilts, p. 325.

izing that gay men are dying in droves and that neither the disease nor its economic consequences can be isolated from the straight community, we can see why a "respectable" and "responsible" group such as the GMHC could succeed where others might fail. New York's education or housing department or a well-financed teaching hospital might resist serving as educators, housers, or caregivers to those with or at risk of AIDS. But the GMHC could take on these roles because it would not be attracting a *new* stigma (it clearly being a group of homosexuals), it already had the health risks of contacts with seropositive people and understood them well, and it would not be spending money on AIDS that "should" have gone to something else. The organization would be vulnerable to the natural shocks of social life that attach to every collective effort, and, given its gay membership cause, it would be somewhat more vulnerable to them than, say, the Red Cross would be. But the specific vulnerabilities of stigma, risk, and cost that we have identified would not overwhelm the group. For the Red Cross, these drawbacks were substantial enough that it initially denied that the infectious agent could be transmitted through blood transfusions or blood products and felt it necessary to avoid publicizing the fact that it was providing ambulance services and home-nursing training to AIDS patients and their lovers.[7]

The experience of the GMHC suggests that new organizations dealing with AIDS will be required to adapt a fairly bureaucratic structure if they are to succeed and will need to be able to interact with sophisticated institutions such as foundations, local government, and power brokers. As obvious as this may sound, it apparently did not occur to the AIDS Institute when it wondered why minority groups were not responding to

7. At least this is how we interpret the extremely circumspect interview material we obtained regarding ambulance services and training. We also found that it took a great deal of effort even to get an interview with the Red Cross, and then it had to be with a public relations person rather than the medical personnel involved with AIDS. The Red Cross's stance on blood is documented in Chapter 2. Interviews with the GMHC were easy to obtain and were very open and helpful. As noted earlier, one-quarter of our interviews in New York City were difficult to obtain and were hostile.

its offers of funds ("requests for proposals"). The gay male community of New York City had the necessary resources to establish a durable and effective organization to give care and counsel to homosexual PWAs, to try to protect their civil liberties, and to some extent even to support research. Many members of the community were affluent, well connected, and equipped with organizational skills. They were so well connected that it is not even clear that they had to respond to requests for proposals; it is likely that the fund givers sought *them* out. By contrast, these critical resources were not available to impoverished communities. In addition, the GMHC, perhaps alone, could undertake the politically explosive task of education among male homosexuals. To gay men it was seen as credible, informed, and very concerned. Government agencies such as the Department of Education and voluntary organizations such as the churches were none of these. To concerned agencies such as the AIDS Institute or private foundations, the GMHC was the ideal group to handle education, and it received substantial sums from these sources (though substantial only in relative terms; we believe that a ten- to hundred-fold increase in education efforts early on would have had a very substantial impact on the spread of the disease).

As a service-oriented organization, GMHC offers many different types of services to its clientele, which includes not only white, affluent gay men but also white women, blacks, Hispanics, and IVDUs.[8] In 1983 a "Buddy Program" was initiated to give each PWA a special friend to help him or her buy groceries, pick up prescriptions, and so on. The financial-services division was started in 1983 to help people receive benefits that they were entitled to. Recreational services were offered in 1983, to give PWAs exercise and the will to continue living. The earliest program, the education and prevention program, has grown to include the hotline for AIDS, AIDS-prevention literature, public speaking, graphic design, community outreach, and the AIDS nutritional training program. GMHC was the first volunteer agency allowed to distribute AIDS educational information at all post offices in New York. The public-

---

8. The breakdown is approximately 50 percent white gay men; 25 percent blacks and Hispanics; 15 percent white women; and 10 percent IVDUs.

policy and the political-advocacy programs started in 1986. Finally, unlike most volunteer organizations, GMHC created a public relations office in 1985 to centralize contact with the media. The establishment of this office has reportedly helped the organization to receive free advertisement for its services to the community.

Today, GMHC can be regarded as a very successful, large, nonprofit, voluntary organization. Its growth and legitimacy were further secured when the city government decided to collaborate with the organization, and when the organization decided to devote some of its resources to the black and Hispanic IVDU population. In 1986 and 1987 GMHC signed contracts with the Division of AIDS Programs Services of the New York City Department of Health under which it was to receive sums amounting to $600,000. By 1988 GMHC had become the largest nongovernmental AIDS organization in the country and the world with a staff of fifty-five paid individuals and over fourteen hundred volunteers, of which straight and lesbian women represent an increasing minority. It spends an annual budget of over $7 million. GMHC's budget would probably amount to over $30 million if the input value of that massive pool of volunteer labor were accounted for.

One final question that the organizational history of GMHC raises is why a large gay male organization did not appear in California as it did in New York. Shilts suggests that the gay community in San Francisco is more politically influential than in New York, and politicians there have to take gay concerns into account when making policy proposals. Additionally, the gay movement tends to follow the grass-roots type in California, but in New York a distinctive "top-down" model predominates, where gay men are less united and "gay political leaders thrive[d] more on the favors of public officials" and the media.[9] Shilts, however, does not notice that New York gay men had to deal with a centralized and slow response to the epidemic on the part of state and local government, whereas in San Francisco funds and programs were much faster to come and the overall approach was more decentralized. A large, bureaucratized organization was much more needed in New York if gay leaders

9. Shilts, pp. 340–341.

wanted to get education and prevention campaigns going; it was less essential in San Francisco, and as a consequence that city's response appears to be more flexible.

Before turning to San Francisco, let us briefly note another initiative on the part of the gay community that has been very successful. The New Haven, Connecticut, AIDS project is an example of an IVDU problem being incorporated into a largely gay white male AIDS program. In 1983, two years into the epidemic, a group of gay men in New Haven set up the AIDS Project New Haven (APNH) as a resource for the gay community. It received no funds from the city, and even five years later most of its money came from the New Haven gay community. Yet by the fall of 1987 it was fielding six part-time outreach workers and had 150 part-time volunteers. Not until then did the city hire its first three outreach workers. That fall APNH received a grant of $7,000 from the state, but none from the city.

The PWA population of New Haven is now coming primarily from IVDUs from the minority community. Although APNH was initially oriented toward a gay constituency, it tooks its resources, including its white outreach workers, into the minority community. In addition to outreach, the most difficult task with IVDUs , the organization attempts to do educational work. For example, it fought a six-month battle with the state transportation department and the state health department to allow APNH to put posters in buses warning of AIDS. Neither state agency appeared to consider AIDS education a legitimate part of its responsibilities.[10]

THE SHANTI PROJECT

In many ways the San Francisco Shanti Project resembles the GMHC of New York City: gay men originally, then hundreds of other volunteers, providing a wide range of services for persons with AIDS, initially with funds raised largely in the gay community and then with municipal, state, and finally federal funds. In a society that squanders its public health monies in a welter of contradictory priorities and rewards

10. Daniel Waterman, "Tracks of the Disease."

to doctors and the drug and medical-equipment industries, voluntary services such as these stand out as the best of our efforts. Technically, the Shanti Project existed before the AIDS epidemic, but for all practical purposes it, like the GMHC, was designed for the epidemic.

In other respects, however, the contrast between the Shanti Project and GMHC is a striking reflection of the distinct cultures of the two cities. The California culture of mysticism, community, and vulnerability to cultlike loyalties has left its mark here. Though it is apparently very effective, Shanti has not been a smooth-running bureaucracy like the GMHC; it was shaken by a scandal in 1988. Both organizations bear the distinctive mark of AIDS: there are charges that minorities and drug users have been neglected. But the Shanti Project's scandal has been, at least temporarily, somewhat disabling. After its meteoric rise to worldwide prominence it was faced by serious charges of corruption, sexual favoritism, and cultlike leadership. These problems now seem to have been overcome with the departure of its leader, bought off by a handsome settlement from the project. Nothing is easy for organizations dealing with AIDS.

The Shanti Project was formed in the late 1970s in Berkeley, California, across the bay from San Francisco, to provide counseling to people dying of cancer. In 1978 Jim Geary joined the organization as a volunteer. He had just lost his job as a masseur at a famous bathhouse that began catering to the "leather" crowd of homosexual men in San Francisco. Before that he had been a hospital orderly, empathic and hard working, loving and warm, a California natural. When gay men began dying of the new disease, the Shanti Project began servicing them, and the group soon moved to San Francisco to be closer to the gay population and also to be eligible for funds being made available by the liberal city government. Geary was by now the head of the organization and appointed his friends to the board of directors. Soon they were concentrating solely on AIDS patients.

Shanti was in the right place at the right time, and it was sorely needed. Private donations and government funds increased, and the organization expanded to provide a variety of counseling services to patients and their lovers and their families, living quarters, shopping and housekeeping services, and a substantial in-house training program. By 1988 its budget was $3 million, with $1.1 million from the city. It housed thirty to forty people with AIDS, trained and deployed 270 volunteer counselors offering practical support to PWAs, and even sent counselors to the principal AIDS hospital, San Francisco General, to help newly diagnosed PWA, cope with their illness. It pioneered many effective AIDS services and was copied throughout the world. Along with the GMHC, it was an example of organizational success in the frightening new world of AIDS.

It still is a success by any reasonable measure, despite the developments that began in early 1988. But Shanti's history since then illustrates the vulnerability of voluntary service organizations. Early in 1988 rumors spread that accused Geary of "sexual harassment, discrimination against women, Jews, and other minorities, nepotism and of assembling a board of directors totally subservient to him,"[11] as one Charles Linebarger put it in the gay paper, the *Bay Area Reporter*. The rumors had been around for some years—Randy Shilts was quoted as saying he had heard them in 1983, but the organization seemed to be doing its job and his newspaper was not particularly interested in pursuing the matter. Nor was anyone else for a long time.

Finally, the complaints of some thirty staff members forced the city's Human Rights Commission (HRC) to investigate systematic discrimination. The commission proceeded gingerly, it would seem; the Shanti Project, after all, was receiving $1.1 million from the city, and in the national field of AIDS care it was as prominent as San Francisco's cable cars. The commission declined to take any investigative action on a number of the subsequent complaints that emerged during the investigation, on the grounds that they were not specified in the original complaint (though it spoke out on other matters not so specified). The commission then turned these over to an internal review committee of the

11. Charles Linebarger, "Scandal at Shanti." We will draw from this article and a subsequent unpublished manuscript by Linebarger, "Scandal Surfaces at the Shanti Project; But Why Was It Kept Secret for So Long?," as well as stories by various authors from the *Bay Area Reporter* (dates listed in the bibliography). We are grateful to Paul Johnston of Yale University for supplying this and other material.

Board (the Board which Geary was accused of stacking with friends and showering with junkets).

Extensive interviews and quotes in the press seem to bear out most of the charges; the sexual harassment is reported in explicit detail, and Geary changed the policy that "no volunteer will engage in a sexual relationship with a Shanti client" to apply only to those with whom there is "a direct ongoing professional relationship." Numerous top staff people were summarily discharged, reportedly after disagreeing with Geary on these and on financial matters. Geary was making $73,000 a year, and his former roommate, the chief financial officer, who had no financial training, was getting much more than others with master's degrees in accounting or finance.

However, the Human Rights Commission determined that many of the charges fell "beyond its jurisdiction"; sexual harassment was not brought up in the original complaint, it said, and nepotism (the favoritism shown to Geary's roommates and close friends) was not a city violation. The HRC filed a formal complaint based only on discrimination. The record of the investigation itself was never made public. No specific charges were brought against Geary; the commission and Shanti's internal review board reached an agreement with him—he would resign and collect a sum of $73,000 over two years in return for a guarantee that the findings of both the HRC and the internal review committee would be sealed. He had threatened to sue, and Shanti officials explained that it would cost more than $73,000 in legal fees to handle the matter in court. The settlement, then, was the best that could be obtained, they said.

Geary left on October 15, 1988, but meanwhile the number of volunteers had dropped by 50 percent in August and September, city funds had been withheld, and donations from individuals were down by $120,000 from the previous year (they totaled $1 million, or one-third of the budget). But the Shanti Project was not seriously hurt and appears to be recovering fast, and for good reason: it is desperately needed. There are other direct client-service organizations in the Bay Area, three of which provide close to $1 million each in direct services to PWAs.[12]

12. The AIDS Emergency Fund, with one full-time and one part-time employee, planned to dispense $900,000 in 1989; the San Francisco AIDS Foundation spends

Shanti, spending about $2.4 million on direct services, is clearly pre-eminent in the struggle to service PWAs. The city provides only 40 percent of its budget; it thus draws into the city's health care system 60 percent of Shanti's budget, funds that come from contributions (33 percent) and grants, benefits, bequests, and sales and fees (27 percent). Shanti remains a success story.

The GMHC and the Shanti Project had moderate to high hurdles to overcome in gaining organizational legitimacy and effectiveness because they were dealing with AIDS and using largely gay, lesbian, or bisexual volunteers. But our third case study, ADAPT, had an even higher hurdle: its clients were intravenous drug users and largely black or Hispanic. Whereas the GMHC and Shanti had the resources of the gay community to draw upon, ADAPT had none. It was difficult for it even to set up an office, and while its board members were largely professionals, they were not prominent ones or experienced in fundraising or managing organizations. Half were ex-addicts. ADAPT's story, then, reveals a quite different aspect of succeeding in the AIDS disaster: how does a group get the resources even to try to get its program on the official agenda? Teaching IVDUs to use condoms and bleach was not a priority for city officials as counseling, homemaking, housing, and the like were in the case of the GMHC and Shanti. In fact, at one time or another the goals of ADAPT were illicit and close to illegal in the city's view. The burden of AIDS for organizations is dramatically revealed by ADAPT's story.

ADAPT: GETTING ON THE AGENDA

In the United States public health is as much a political and moral issue as it is a professional one. The stigma attached to AIDS makes it hard for organizations to add tasks related to AIDS to their

---

$1 million; Eighteenth Street Services (drug-related) spends $256,000; Family Link (help to PWAs relatives), $106,000; Open Hand (meals for PWAs), $920,000; and Coming Home Organization (financial services), $80,000. These and several smaller organizations are described in the *Bay Area Reporter*, December 8, 1988, along with an account of Shanti's recovery.

programs. This is well illustrated by the case of ADAPT, and it is force-fully brought out by Cherni L. Gillman, of the Narcotic and Drug Research organization in New York City. We will draw liberally from her work as well as from an interview with ADAPT's executive director, Yolanda Serrano, and from press reports.[13]

The Association for Drug Abuse Prevention and Treatment was set up initially in the 1970s to pressure for greater treatment capacity for the city's drug-rehabilitation centers. For years the board of directors was the largest group in the organization, sometimes the only membership; most of the directors were middle-class professionals such as lawyers, doctors, and health care workers, and about half of them had been addicts. The group represented an example of a tiny but vital part of health services in the United States — the other-regarding, community-service, and advocacy groups, made up of volunteers with only occasionally a poorly paid, hard-working executive, groups that try to address the mani-fold human problems of our fragmented, politicized health sector. Thou-sands of them can exist in a large city, with life spans of a few years, and occasionally one has an impact.

ADAPT stopped meeting in 1983, for no apparent reason, according to its current director, Yolanda Serrano. But former members began to notice that IVDUs were dying of the new disease, AIDS. Serrano, who had been working in drug-rehabilitation clinics for some time, and other concerned workers decided to resurrect ADAPT rather than start a new group to cope with this new problem.

In 1985, under its new mission, ADAPT board members and volun-teers went into the streets to encourage addicts to use bleach kits and condoms and to enter treatment programs. One of the things that made ADAPT so successful was that it could quickly get people into one of the very few methadone treatment programs. The volunteers were able to do this by contacting all the programs to see when a slot was likely to be available. Otherwise, the typical wait was six to nine months, during which time the habit would get worse and the user's resolve weaker. The

13. Gillman, "Genesis of New York City's Experimental Needle Exchange Program."

program also worked at educating community groups and government agencies; in particular, it visited and brought pressure to bear upon the local and state prison system, which had its own share of illicit sex and drug abuse and the mistreatment of inmates with AIDS. ADAPT's budget for 1985 was a tiny $1,500, part of it contributed by the board members.

Gillman argues that the organization knew that because of its tiny size and the vulnerability of its directors —who could lose their professional licenses for distributing or advocating the distribution of needles or even bleach for cleaning needles —it could hardly make a dent in the estimated population of 200,000 IVDUs in New York City. But it was, in Gillman's words, engaged in "agenda setting." It was trying to get the issue of clean needles and AIDS on the agenda of public organizations concerned with drug abuse, and particularly on the mayor's agenda. Otherwise, nothing would happen.

The task was awesome. The organization had to demonstrate that it was possible to reach IVDUs and get them to use sterilized equipment. For this, they had to go to the "shooting galleries," abandoned buildings where illicit drug dealing, injection, and prostitution frequently take place. For a couple of dollars an IVDU can rent the paraphernalia used for injection (needles, syringes, heater, cotton, cup of water, elastic band), and dozens of users can share the equipment. Drugs are easy to buy, sterile needles are not, and if any needles are available for sale they may be nonsterile ones packaged and sold as sterile. Bleach is not often available, nor even a source of running water for rinsing bleach from the needle or syringe. An addict in intense need for a fix may not want to take the time to clean the "works." As Gillman notes, "there are chilling stories of addicts sharing needles, starting with the healthiest looking person first and ending with the individual who appears sickest."

ADAPT board members, volunteers, and director Serrano gained such acceptance in the shooting galleries over time that the addicts would allow television crews to come with Serrano and film their behavior. A reporter quoted a recovering addict, speaking of Serrano: "She's like the Avon lady [with her bleach kits and condoms]. At first you think, the lady is *nuts*. She's going into buildings the police won't go near, taking her life into her own hands."[14] (When TV personality Geraldo Rivera accompanied Serrano once, an addict kept playfully stabbing at him with a (presumably infected) needle; Rivera kept jumping back.)[15]

After ADAPT changed its emphasis from encouraging IVDUs to seek treatment to helping them avoid AIDS and avoid spreading it to their sexual partners, workers from New York State's Division of Substance Abuse Services approached the agency to formulate an organized response to the problem. ADAPT applied to the City Department of Health (DOH) for funding. But the DOH refused because the organization was distributing bleach kits and thus "encouraging" addiction. ADAPT persisted. But it needed more than courageous board members and volunteers to visit the mean streets. To be funded ADAPT needed the paraphernalia of bureaucracy—the "organizational works," so to speak, of governmental addicts—and it needed organizational allies.

ADAPT got the support of the Community Service Society (CSS), which works with social-policy and advocacy groups to fight poverty, and the New York Foundation, active in health matters and willing to take risks. These organizations gave ADAPT the help it needed to make the transition to a properly funded, rule-bound organization. The foundation offered staff support and organized a retreat for formulating goals and strategies. ADAPT's efforts would be not only controversial but illegal, and considerable planning and reflection were needed. To write grant proposals it needed personnel policies, accounting procedures, bylaws, an address, office space, a staff, bonds, insurance, a utility account, and a telephone. ADAPT, Gillman notes, had none of these, and CSS and the New York Foundation helped provide them. The organization then could apply for a start-up grant from the Department of Health, now that it had started up. Without these emblems of establishment, ADAPT would have found it impossible to be noticed and to get their issue on the city's agenda. Recall that to some extent the city was looking for organizations that worked in impoverished areas to send at

14. Zoe Carter, "Local Hero: ADAPT and Survive."
15. Gillman, "Genesis of New York City's Experimental Needle Exchange Program."

least token sums to, but these organizations needed the trappings of stability and reliability, such as phone and electric bills, taken for granted by modern officialdom.

The organization was still minuscule by any standards, especially in comparison with the population of 200,000 hard-to-reach IVDUs it meant to serve, when it went once again in late 1986 and early 1987 to the city for funds. But it was needed and funded and began to grow. In 1987, when we visited ADAPT, its far-flung efforts to target several different segments of the minority community were carried out by only three full-time staff members and eight outreach workers (former IVDUs, some still in treatment). It had a grant of $100,000 from the AIDS Institute, its principal source of money, a sum equivalent to less than $10,000 per staff member. The director felt, of course, that much more was needed and had sought more from the AIDS Institute, but most of the funding for the minority communities from the AIDS Institute and the Robert Wood Johnson Foundation had gone to a more conventional program, the Brooklyn AIDS Task Force. Though poor, ADAPT was at least a serious player in the AIDS-prevention area.

Serrano argued that IVDUs can be reached in an educational effort and that ADAPT was reaching them; that many organizations in the minority community, such as the social clubs, could be used for education; and that the writers and the stars of the Spanish-language afternoon television dramas, which are very popular, could be persuaded to include AIDS in their shows. The older Hispanic population, she said, engaged in massive denial regarding AIDS; techniques would have to be developed to reach the young and the vulnerable. All this would take much more money than the AIDS Institute was willing to provide.

Shortly after ADAPT had received the blessings and some money from the AIDS Institute, City Health Commissioner Stephen Joseph announced that it was "the most credible community action group on drug abuse in New York City."[16] By then, January 1988, fourteen persons, most of them professionals, were on the board, the staff included fifty volunteers and fifteen full- or part-time workers, and the organiza-

16. Lambert, "Drug Group to Offer Free Needles."

tion had received international recognition. By any standards it was still minuscule, but in a city where AIDS agendas were virtually invisible, even a tiny organization could fancy setting an agenda.

But getting on the agenda, even with the help of the New York Foundation and the Community Service Society, was not easy. Aside from the mean streets there were ideological and political problems to overcome. As we have noted before, two groups may prefer to countenance death by AIDS rather than "encourage" drug abuse: those whose professional lives are devoted to discouraging drug abuse, and those whose religious or conservative political positions require putting morality ahead of lives. ADAPT was to confront both.

The idea of distributing free, sterile needles to addicts was initially proposed by City Health Commissioner David Sencer in 1985, but public prosecutors were opposed to it and Mayor Koch let the matter drop.[17] Sencer was replaced by Dr. Stephen Joseph, who proposed a limited experiment in 1986, which the mayor approved. The plan called for sending mobile vans to areas where drugs were used and making counselors available to urge addicts to enroll in treatment programs. Ironically, the program would have to be very small or it would stimulate too much demand for treatment; the waiting list for treatment was already very long. Indeed, as noted, one of the things that made ADAPT credible to the IVDUs was that it was able to get people into treatment programs quickly by being very persistent and working very hard at finding the odd open slot.

The city's controversial needle plan was widely opposed by many and was successively scaled down, from serving 6,000 IVDUs to only 200. These 200 would be required to undertake counseling in order to get a clean needle, and there had to be a "control group" of 200 who got counseling only. As limited as the program would be for preventing AIDS, it was a substantial increase in resources devoted to the problem. The new version was submitted in November 1987 to the State Health Commissioner, Dr. David Axelrod, who did not rule on the request over the next fourteen months. ADAPT decided to force the issue and in

17. Bruce Lambert, "Drug Group to Offer Free Needles," *op. cit.*

January 1988 announced that it was considering a civil-disobedience action: distributing free needles on its own.

It was a courageous act. Board members, Gillman points out, were certain that they would be arrested for distributing needles, and those who had histories of drug use would face harsh sentences. Some board members might jeopardize their professional licenses. Certainly, the existence of the organization could be jeopardized if it carried out the program. But because of the announcement that it was under consideration and Serrano's statement that she was willing to go to jail (it was that important to her to try to stem AIDS deaths among addicts and their sexual partners and children), the proposed plan, languishing in the office of the State Health Commissioner, got on the agenda once again, this time with a vocal, credible, and properly bureaucratized voluntary organization pushing it. But the city struck back.

The Department of Health froze ADAPT's operating money and did not reimburse ADAPT for any of its city-related expenditures for three months. It was also able to shut down ADAPT's offices for two days. Mayor Koch, who had approved the original plan for distributing needles in 1986, now threatened to arrest any members caught distributing needles. But the city was unexpectedly outflanked and embarrassed by Governor Cuomo and Commissioner Axelrod, who now found it expedient to approve the city's own needle-distribution plan, which they had been pondering for so long. The city was then saved by its special narcotics prosecutor, Sterling Johnson, who said the program that Stephen Joseph had whittled down from 6,000 to 200, and that the mayor had earlier approved, was illegal. He announced, "The Health Commissioner can designate whoever he wants to have needles, but you cannot authorize somebody to take a legal instrument and use it for an illegal purpose." Johnson added to the reporter: "I think that's stopped them in their tracks."[18] It did. The State Health Commissioner acknowledged that the plan would not work without the cooperation of law-enforcement personnel.

But Commissioners Axelrod and Joseph continued their efforts, and

18. Barron, "Health Chief Sees Obstacle to AIDS Needle Plan."

six months later they announced that the local law-enforcement officials would cooperate with the plan since it was an "authorized research plan." It had not been removed from the agenda, but by now the plan was quite ridiculous. IVDUs would have to travel to lower Manhattan, the seat of all city and state authority and bureaucracy, register at the courthouse (under the watchful eye of TV news cameras), accept counseling and *no* free needle if so assigned, or, if they were put in the group that also got a free new needle, accept counseling and journey back for a new needle the next time they needed a fix if they happened to have let others use theirs. As the president of Phoenix House, the largest drug-free program in New York, and one not particularly in favor of free needle programs or methadone programs without counseling, pointed out, these are the most disordered people in society; to expect them "to register and appear regularly flies in the face of what we know."[19]

The experimental program began in November 1988; only a handful of addicts braved extensive press coverage. Shortly thereafter it was deemed a failure, as it was bound to be, but the issue of needle distribution had made its way onto the agenda. Once there it produced the predictable outcry from law-enforcement officials, the Catholic Church, the minority community, and the City Council itself.

The head of the black and Hispanic caucus on the City Council declared: "The City is sending the wrong message when it distributes free needles to drug addicts while we are trying to convince our children to say no to drugs." Black officials opposed to the program included U.S. Representative Charles Rangel, Manhattan Borough President (and, in 1990, Mayor) David Dinkins, the head of the largest drug treatment program in Brooklyn and member of President Reagan's AIDS commission, Dr. Beny J. Primm, several religious leaders, and the special narcotics prosecutor, Sterling Johnson.

The reasons for resistance to the program are varied but clear. For example, there is a great deal of violent crime associated with drug abuse. As one respondent asked Gillman in an interview, "Do victims of violent crime care whether their mugger gets sick and dies of AIDS?"

19. Peter Kerr, "Experts Find Fault in New AIDS Plan."

David Dinkins felt that the needle-exchange program promotes tolerance of drug use; Beny Primm thought that free needles are only a cheap
and ineffective substitute for more serious and elaborate drug-prevention
programs and lessen the resolve to provide such programs; the special
prosecutor thought that it encouraged the crime of drug abuse; Congressman Rangel implied that racism was at work, charging that instead
of making people strong enough to enable them to resist drugs we give
needles to them to keep them in "little cells of despair and poverty";
and the Reverend Calvin Butts, pastor of the Abyssinian Baptist Church
in Harlem, simply stated: "I am not in favor of cooperating with evil."

The Catholic Church was opposed. Cardinal O'Connor accused the
city of "dragging down the standards of all society." Surgeon General
Everett Koop explained his disapproval in concrete terms: "You'll give
out the needles and never see these people again." The *New York Post*
editorialized against it, arguing that we should not lose our "moral bear-
ings." And the New York City Council voted unanimously to end the
nine-month experimental program after one month of operation and three
months of bombardment from powerful interests. An editorial in *The
Nation* commented on all this opposition: "The conservative fantasy of
how people ought to behave is not worth dying for."[20]

Through it all, ADAPT survived and even prospered, and perhaps in
part as a response to all its trouble (but to many other pressures, of
course), the city is at last taking more than a token step in expanding
methadone clinics. It is not easy for an organization to tackle any part of
the AIDS problem, so engulfed is the problem in moral, ideological,
and political agendas, so expensive, and so threatening in so many ways.
But to address the problems of AIDS in combination with those of drug
abuse and poverty is especially difficult. We should not be surprised that
there are so few drug or community organizations that could incorporate

20. The quotes regarding opposition to the program, assembled by Gillman, can
be found in the following news stories: "Council Calls for End to Free-Needles
Plan"; Dicker and Bollinger, "Top Narc Takes Shot at AIDS Needle Plan"; Evans
and Santangelo, "O'C Blasts Addict Plan"; Lambert, "Ethics and Needles"; London, "Free Needles?"; "Realism on AIDS"; and Ryan, "Give People Hope, Not
Drugs."

the AIDS problem into their plan of action. In fact, ADAPT is not an example of an existing organization that added AIDS to its agenda. This tiny organization was quiescent until it was transformed by the epidemic into a quite different one.

The ADAPT story reinforces other, more general themes of community action. Minority organizations need assistance starting up, given the criteria for competence and accountability that government bureaucracies and even most private foundations insist upon. If there were more groups like the Community Service Society and even the New York Foundation, more community groups might survive to do the hands-on work that is required. The fears of the minority community about encouraging drug use by distributing free needles (or sexual promiscuity by condom advertising) cannot be dismissed; these people bear the brunt of these problems. Addressing their fears will take a lot more contact with the desperate segments of the minority communities and more exposure to their problems than nonminority politicians and business and industrial elites have at present. High-ranking Catholics can be expected to make unqualified statements about just saying no, but since AIDS and poverty are eating away at their fastest-growing constituency —the Hispanic population—perhaps they could be made to see that moralizing about these problems will eventually work against them. Perhaps city officials should work out ways whereby the liberal elements in the church can quietly promote education and tolerance, even though the "alliance" between Cardinal O'Connor and Mayor Koch did not appear to be constructive in this regard.[21]

Finally, ADAPT's work indicates the intricate web that AIDS is caught in—virtually every major social problem is worsened by this epidemic, making solutions to these problems—homelessness, alcoholism, drug abuse, teenage pregnancies, single-parent families, unemployment and unemployability, tuberculosis, syphilis and other sexually transmitted diseases, and crime—all the more difficult.

21. See O'Connor and Koch, *His Eminence and Hizzoner: A Candid Exchange.*

8 AIDS AND EXISTING ORGANIZATIONS

Most organizational analysis utilizes one of two approaches, neither of which seems appropriate for analyzing the response of existing organizations to the AIDS crisis. In the first, the "macro" perspective, the challenges facing an organization are to make the proper long-term strategic choices (which market to emphasize, whether to centralize or decentralize the structure, whether to contract out or not, and so on), to acquire the proper form of leadership, since leadership should vary with the environment and the organizational structure, and to make the proper links to the environment. Strategic matters of this sort were important in the AIDS crisis, but they were decided by political authorities rather than by the heads of service organizations. The AIDS Institute, for example, owed both its existence and its mandate to centralize its activities to Governor Cuomo. Our national AIDS policy—a policy of waging war on illicit drugs and illegitimate sex, rather than of medicalizing the disease and trying to minimize its harm—is also a strategic choice. But it too is not an "organizational" response but a political choice made—perhaps not even consciously made—at the highest levels.

Among the organizations that would be expected to respond to AIDS in a more concrete way, such as the hospitals, community groups, and the blood banks, we do not detect any gross strategic "mistakes" that could have been rectified by choosing an alternative strategy that was available. For example, we suspect that it was fear of being associated with stigmatized groups that led the blood banks to deny the need for risk-group screening for so long and then to refuse to use the available blood test for the core antibody of hepatitis B. Nor do we see any particularly powerful leadership problems; organizations cannot rely upon getting superhuman leaders, and none of the leaders, including elected officials, was incompetent. Jim Geary of the Shanti Project was certainly inefficient and perhaps corrupt, but he got the organization going, and if, as charged, he proceeded to use it for his own illegitimate ends, it recovered quickly once he left.

The second approach to organizational studies, the "micro" perspective, is concerned with employee motivation, morale, job structuring, surveillance and supervision, skill levels, supervisory leadership, and so on. There were problems of this sort among the organizations we studied, but we do not believe that they went beyond the normal difficulties of providing for good incentives, better morale, more appropriately skilled people, and the like. Burnout is probably more frequent in AIDS organizations than in other service organizations, and the pay has been low, but these are not likely to be important contributors to what we have described as a massive organizational failure.

Both major perspectives and several other variants, such as network analysis, population and ecology, Marxist and ethnological perspectives, take for granted something that should always be problematical. They assume that organizations have solved the basic problems of multiple missions or mandates, conflicting goals, goal distortion, and unauthorized usage or the exploitation of organizational resources.

The third perspective, which we have been using, makes no such assumption. Instead, it assumes that the goals of the organization are only weakly defined (patient care, yes, but perhaps not all patients), that goals are subject to internal contradictions (a research goal that requires the study of patients may conflict with the goal of patient care), that personal ideologies and beliefs cannot always be set aside (so personnel discriminate against minorities or cannot bring themselves to provide safe-sex education), and even that there is a good deal of chance, accident, and unanticipated interaction that may deflect organizations from goals truly subscribed to by everyone.

In this view organizations are very imperfect and even recalcitrant "tools" in the hands of the authorities who oversee them or the leaders who run them. Organizations will fail much of the time to achieve their official purpose, which is always stated in misleadingly clear, rational terms. Some challenges, such as AIDS, may be so difficult that they will (1) interfere with other legitimate programs, (2) provoke denial, flight, or refusal to deal with the challenge, (3) lead to segregation of the tasks and thus to inaction, (4) distort or deflect the very purposes of the organization, or (5) even disable or destroy parts of the organization or its legitimate purposes.

Which of these failures or defenses against the challenge is invoked depends on the setting of the organization (a highly politicized context, for example, may lead to flight), its size and strength (large, strong organizations may be bogged down by segregation and inaction more easily than small ones are), its resource vulnerability (if it draws heavily from an ideological community, as a church may, it cannot easily resist that ideology), the source of key personnel (can they resist association with a stigmatized population?), or unexpected interactions (diverting resources to cope with a challenge may unintentionally increase the vulnerability of the population it is meant to serve). We have found evidence of all these mechanisms.

Early in the post–World War II history of organizational analysis there was a good deal of concern with the problem of distortion of goals and goal displacement (as when the means utilized becomes more important than the original goal and displace it, or when rules are implacably defended even though they are not appropriate to changing situations and the rules become the goals). It has been designated the "exposé" tradition: exposing the failure of organizations to pursue their legitimate goals. It is now more or less out of favor, as theorists, assuming that the goals are in place and drive behavior, have focused on the macro issues of major strategies or the micro issues of motivation and efficiency. Here we are interested in more than exposés, though they are certainly necessary. Instead, we will be examining the *context* in which the organizations operate, the internal and external *interest groups* that seek to use it for their own ends, and the very *limited degree of rationality* that is possible when information is incomplete, preferences unclear, control of subordinates uncertain, and unexpected interactions possible. Ours, in a phrase, is a "recalcitrant-tool" view of organizations.[1]

We think it is the appropriate perspective for the AIDS crisis. It seems to us that what is most relevant is not an organization's direction (strategic studies, leadership) or the energies of its employees (the dominant micro concern) but the success of the organization in warding off everpresent external and internal threats. In the tool view, the problems of concern are outside the normal range of the other two views; the problems arise because latent, endemic organizational contradictions surface from within and because outside interests impose constraints and goals that sometimes cannot even be acknowledged. Even assuming that they are not one of the problems, organizational leaders often lack the mechanisms to solve them or even the symbols to disguise their failure.

If an organization is challenged by a new problem, like AIDS, and that problem is sufficiently difficult or affects a number of internal and external groups, there is a good chance that the organization will fail to achieve its mandated goals. The mechanisms that prevent distortion of its goals or improper use of its resources may not be strong enough for the new challenge. It is as if the organization lacked sufficiently effective "immune responses." The interests that are normally held in check surface, almost like "opportunistic infections" in the body; an organization's goals will be distorted or unmet, its operation may be tainted by discrimination, and its response may be one of flight or inaction. Organizations are always vulnerable to such "opportunistic infections," but they have mechanisms—defenses—to prevent goal distortion, inaction, and discrimination. Furthermore, superordinate organizations, including organizations in the legal system, have such mechanisms and enforce them in the organizations over which they have jurisdiction. It is our argument that the uniqueness of AIDS makes it very easy to overwhelm

1. For a discussion of the exposé tradition, see Perrow, *Complex Organizations*, pp. 159–164. See the entire book for a statement of the view that organizations are tools and that investigating the uses they are put to should be the central thrust of organizational theory. For application to human service organizations, see Perrow, "Demystifying Organizations."

these defenses. Only in the most favorable of circumstances—in a city such as San Francisco, for example, with its powerful gay community, a few minorities or IVDUs, more integrated health system, and a culture of caring—can organizations surmount the challenge, and even then not fully.

There is a danger of pushing too far the analogy between the HIV infection overwhelming the immune system of the human body and the disabling of organizational "defenses." The effects of ideology, stratification, the power structure, and human agency in its many forms make any biological analysis suspect. But the usefulness of the analogy is that it demands a *system-level* analysis, one that examines the interaction of many components and many levels. In our analysis we will examine the context or setting of the organization, the interest groups within and without the organization, and the unexpected interactions that can occur given the limited degree of control (or "rationality") that any of the actors have.

ORGANIZATIONAL RESPONSES TO AIDS

Think of an organization with ongoing programs that could be utilized for persons with AIDS (PWAs). The organization could be a hospital that treats people, a social service organization offering help with personal and financial problems, a housing authority, and so on. AIDS is a problem that the organization should deal with just as it deals with, for example, diabetes, unemployment, or lack of education.

When confronted with the new problem (a PWA, for example, or just someone seeking information), the organization can respond in a variety of ways. The outcome affects both the existing programs—health education in the schools, for example—and the AIDS component in particular. Figure 8-1 schematically represents the responses we shall illustrate, with a line or two representing the ongoing programs encountering AIDS, the consequences of the encounter, and a brief reference to the examples we shall give.

Figure 8-1. *The impact of AIDS on existing organizations*

Pattern	Ongoing program encounters AIDS	Organizational outcomes	Examples from text
A	1 → A ← 2 →	AIDS incorporated; programs enriched	Village Nursing Home
B	1 — (A) — 2 —	AIDS handled; other programs suffer	Diversion of medical research; STD clinics suffer; hospital emergency rooms
C	1 — (A) — 2 —	Refusal to deal with AIDS; denial, flight	Federal and local delays; blood screening; methadone clinics; Housing Authority in New York
D	1 — 2 — (A) →	AIDS segregated into task force; little done	Initial response of New York State and City; Social Security Administration office
E	1 — (A) ↘	Organizational purpose distorted or deflected	Schools; hospital misdiagnosis; CDC research lab; Catholic Archdiocese shelter
F	1 — (A)	Unit or its purpose disabled or destroyed	Hospital special team; CDC research lab; minority families of PWAs

Note: Organizations created as a response to AIDS, such as GMHC and APNH, or completely remade by events related to the disease, such as ADAPT and the Shanti Project, are not assessed here.

AIDS Is Incorporated into Ongoing Programs

The first case is the successful one. The normal programs of the organization are handled in such a way that the AIDS problem (service to PWAs, education, or whatever) is incorporated into the existing work of the organization, and the existing programs may even be enriched as a result. This model presumes that organizational elites will work to secure additional resources for this additional task. We would expect smaller organizations with the potential for growth to be likely candidates for incorporating AIDS successfully. These small, growth-prone organizations are not as "exposed" to the problems of multiple constituencies or multiple, conflicting goals as are federal or local governments, say, or long-standing voluntary, nonprofit, or for-profit hospitals and clinics. Another explanation would argue that it was precisely because of inaction or delays on the part of large, established organizations, that smaller organizations, not so worried about the stigma of AIDS, could mobilize the financial and volunteer resources to provide the required services. Existing community-based or self-help organizations may also incorporate AIDS in a desperate attempt to provide services in the midst of a full-scale epidemic.

Remarkably enough, we could not find a single convincing example of any *major* organization that took on AIDS, so to speak, without question and without problems. The organizations we examined in interviews and in our literature search (other than those formed to deal with AIDS, like GMHC or ADAPT) have all taken on other problems and diseases, secured the necessary resources, and incorporated these other problems into their programs. But not AIDS. There are probably many organizations that have done so that we did not find in the literature or our interviews—for example, many hospitals that have treated AIDS patients without goal distortion or other failures in its operation. But even among the hospitals where we interviewed we found resistance, denial, false diagnosis, and the like.

Methadone clinics may have been able to incorporate AIDS programs into drug treatment programs if they had been able to expand their case loads and educational services when the demand for treatment rose. This would appear to have been in the interests of everyone; AIDS would be stemmed, and addicts brought into treatment, for a fraction of the cost of caring for PWAs or imprisoning addicts for drug abuse or the crimes associated with feeding a drug habit. Demand has long exceeded the supply of places in methadone clinics, with waits of two to six months; the waiting periods rose even further when IVDUs learned about the danger of AIDS and were more disposed to be drawn into treatment. Unfortunately, the necessary funds were not appropriated.

Even attempts to establish "cut-rate," minimalist programs that did little more than keep a register, warn of the AIDS danger, and hand out methadone to those who otherwise would need to purchase heroin proved to be impossible to start. Programs of this sort would be illegal without special federal approval, and that has not been available, though the situation was changing in 1989. The New York State Division of Substance Abuse Services finally established Key Extended Entry Programs (KEEP) that work along these lines. Although some change was noted in 1988, law-enforcement personnel, some drug experts, and most minority community leaders have not allowed programs to be established that did not include expensive full-service counseling, employment, and other services. Many still resist these pared-down programs.[2] AIDS was, in effect, a hostage to the requirement that distribution of the drug methadone be accompanied by a cure for drug dependency, whereas it might have been a means of bringing people into at least some contact with service personnel, reducing the crime associated with feeding a cocaine or heroin habit, and educating drug users about AIDS. The proposal to provide clean needles to reduce the risk of infection was also a hostage; free needles might encourage drug dependency, some drug experts and

---

2. See, for example, the argument by the president of Phoenix House, a full-service, drug-free treatment program, in Michell S. Rosenthal, "Methadone Clone: A Bad Quick Fix." On easing up on the rules specifying treatment for those receiving methadone by federal health agencies in the face of the epidemic, see Altman, "U.S. to Ease Methadone Rules." But a relaxation of rules was not enough for public interest groups in New York. The Coalition for the Homeless, a feisty, effective group of hard-working, poorly paid lawyers and aides, filed a lawsuit to force New York State and City officials to provide drug treatment for all city residents who seek it. See Sara Rimer, "Lawsuit Seeks Drug Treatment on Demand."

many community leaders argued. Just as the threat of nonmarital sex can seem more urgent than the threat of death itself, as when the moral majority opposes the mention of condoms, so has the threat of incomplete treatment or the appearance of condoning intravenous drug use overshadowed the threat of death.

The example of the Village Nursing Home (VNH) in Manhattan is too recent to be considered a successful incorporation of AIDS into an existing organization, but we will nonetheless risk the following preliminary analysis. VNH was a proprietary skilled-nursing facility before it nearly went bankrupt in the mid-1970s. The Lower Manhattan community raised the money to convert VNH into a nonprofit, community-based organization providing geriatric services for the severely impaired elderly. The organization runs a 200-bed facility with a paid staff of over 230, about twelve of whom currently deal with AIDS patients.

VNH's AIDS adventure began in 1986, when the Rockefeller Foundation was approached to fund a specialized AIDS program that would provide much-needed long-term health care. With the financial assistance of many other foundations (amounting to over $750,000), VNH conducted preliminary need-assessment studies, renovated space, trained health care professionals, and acquired equipment. Three types of services have been planned as part of VNH's AIDS program: an adult day-treatment center, a home-care service, and a 200-bed skilled-nursing facility. Only the first of these projects, the day-treatment center, is currently functioning, at a renovated ground-floor space leased from the GMHC. The center now delivers services to fifty AIDS patients referred from New York City hospitals, the GMHC, the AIDS Resource Center, the Community Health Project, or private doctors in the community. Seventy-five percent of VNH's AIDS patients are gay or bisexual males, while IVDUs and female sex partners of IVDUs account for 20 and 5 percent, respectively. It is worth noting that 25 and 20 percent of all these AIDS patients are Hispanics and blacks, respectively. Thus, the composition of the group of patients does not exactly reflect the overall distribution of cases in the city, but it is not nearly as biased toward wealthier groups as the city's major hospital centers. The professional and bureaucratic nature of the organization may be behind this seemingly good record on patient discrimination.

In 1988 the total AIDS budget at VNH reached $1.2 million, with about 85 percent financed by Medicaid. Further involvement of the nonhospital health care industry might ease the burden that AIDS patients now represent for New York City hospitals. New facilities like the VNH or the city's Bailey House, a forty-four-bed facility for homeless PWAs, are only a partial solution to the overcrowding crisis in city hospitals.

As Leonard McNally, VNH's AIDS program director, explained in an interview, the only problem AIDS has made for the organization is the disproportionate increase in the number of staff working in the fundraising and accounting areas. Though it is small, VNH is our one example of an organization that incorporated AIDS into its program without disrupting its existing programs.

In sum, until the past year or so, well into the epidemic, we have seen only one rather small *existing* organization *adding resources* to cope with the new threat of AIDS. There are undoubtedly some large ones and perhaps many small ones, but given the size of the epidemic we would have expected to find many more. Only new groups, primarily started by gay activists or private drug-abuse groups such as ADAPT, have tackled the AIDS problem, but they were formed (or revitalized) for that purpose. Only gradually have state drug-abuse groups in New York, New Jersey, Illinois, and perhaps elsewhere responded with new money and programs within their jurisdiction. The failure to expand methadone clinics in, say, 1984, was an unfortunate missed opportunity.

AIDS Crisis Is Addressed, But Other Programs Suffer

A still benign but unfortunate response is illustrated by panel B in Figure 8-1. Here a lack of new resources plus a commitment or obligation to deal with AIDS means that existing programs suffer as the resources are diverted to AIDS. Initial hardships are fairly commonplace when new demands are made on organizations, but within a year or so the organization's leaders usually manage to secure more funds for the new programs. What distinguishes the AIDS case is not only the delay of years in obtaining new funds but the resentment engendered (and, in one case we will discuss shortly, an unexpected interaction that made things worse).

AIDS drew money from other legitimate pursuits in sufficient volume to be an issue in the Centers for Disease Control from the beginning, in other federal public health agencies, and in many hospitals and other settings. Even when new resources were appropriated, resentment from the champions of other causes may be expected. We were told that medical researchers at the major hospitals and research centers not only resented any diversion of funds to AIDS research but saw the appropriations of large amounts of new money in the past two years as a mortgage on medical research in general. In New York City the hospital bed crisis, due to AIDS, homelessness, tuberculosis, and drug abuse (and interactions among these problems), has meant jammed emergency rooms, AIDS patients crowded into storage rooms, and four-day waits before a cardiac patient can get a regular bed with the appropriate monitoring equipment and nursing. In addition, it has raised the specter of the loss of much-needed jobs for the city when business leaders point to the lack of bed space as a reason for directing their firms to leave, expand elsewhere, or not move to the city.[3]

Public health researcher Nicholas Freudenberg reports one particularly unfortunate outcome of the use of funds allocated for STD programs for AIDS. In the black community, the STD facilities were often the only source of medical care IVDUs had. There was no waiting, no names were required, and little bureaucracy stood between them and medical care. Responding to Freudenberg's survey, STD workers in sev-

3. The hospital-bed crisis is regularly aired, with increasing alarm, in *New York Times* stories. For an account of the current crisis, see Lambert, "Hospital Shortages Hurt Patient Care"; and Lambert, "Outlook Dim for Expanding Health Care."

On the contribution of AIDS to the crisis, see, for example, Lambert, "Concentration of AIDS Cases." The story notes that in 1987 the average public hospital in New England and the South lost over $600,000 on AIDS patients. "Treating AIDS is largely a losing proposition," said the president of the National Public Health and Hospital Institute and author of the study, Dennis P. Andrulis. He did not say what kind of a proposition *not* treating the disease would be.

eral cities said that as money was diverted from the outpatient clinics to (unspecified) AIDS work, they lost contact with the very people who most needed education and help.[4] The adverse effect on non-AIDS care was an unanticipated system interaction.

Refusal, Denial, and Flight

Panel C in Figure 8-1 illustrates the most common of the unfortunate organizational responses to AIDS: refusal to deal with the crisis, denial of its existence, denial of the organization's failures, and in general insulation from the problem. Existing programs just go on; perhaps they are slightly deflected for a time by AIDS problems. We have treated the Koch administration's reported failure to make more than a token response as an example; the federal response is another one. But there are more specific examples.

We have noted that the blood-bank industry for some years refused to screen high-risk groups and to screen for evidence of risk of hepatitis B. Providing safe blood was the industry's mandate; it not only failed to ensure a safe supply, but at first it denied that there was any danger and then later it denied having failed. While screening could mean a decline in donations of blood in general, and by homosexual men in particular (who reportedly already gave much more than any other identifiable group), and a small increase in cost, we suspect that the stigma problem was the biggest reason for the failure to confront the danger—the association of life-giving blood and "diseased homosexual men" was simply too much for the blood industry.

The New York City housing authority provides another example. Normally one would expect the Housing Administration to make a reasonable effort to provide housing for any homeless group suffering from a debilitating, disabling, and deadly disease. Its official job is to look after the housing needs of citizens. With some 25,000 empty or abandoned units in New York City, finding housing for one or two thousand

---

4. Nicholas Freudenberg, "The Politics of AIDS Education." Professor Freudenberg is Director of the Program in Community Health Sciences, City University of New York.

PWAs who had lost their homes should not be an unreasonable challenge for a giant agency. Besides, it has been widely observed that bureaucracies typically make efforts to grow; they should therefore welcome tasks that will bring in more resources. Yet when a consortium of organizations that could deal with AIDS problems was formed in the city, the housing administration withdrew from it, to the consternation of many members. It took a special effort by the mayor, we were told, to get the authority to provide any housing at all for PWAs. Asked why the housing authority was so reluctant to pitch in, a respondent said that the authority was interested in improving the housing stock and the neighborhoods; PWAs do neither.

Even small proposals were resisted, another told us. This respondent, from the City Council, noted that when Manhattan Borough President David Dinkins pressed for expansion of the Human Resources Administration's scattered-site housing program, the HRA resisted. Dinkins and City Council President Andrew Stein wanted it to be increased from fifteen units to twenty. This is a trivial figure considering that there were an estimated 650 homeless PWAs at the time, 1986–1987, but it would be a substantial expansion of the city's existing stock of about fifty units for PWAs. Eventually Dinkins prevailed. Why the resistance? The respondent speculated that the HRA was already overburdened, what with the homeless and other poverty problems; that it was not interested in expanding its organization even though growth would be consistent with its mandate; and that it felt that AIDS should not be its responsibility.

Thus, a pattern of avoidance seems to have existed. Since other major cities, such as Boston, Los Angeles, and San Francisco, had housing programs for PWAs before New York City began to do anything, it appears to be a New York City phenomenon more than an AIDS phenomenon —but we expect that the other cities ran into similar problems, but prevailed. The lack of housing also affects those with tuberculosis, most of whom are poor. Tuberculosis is carried by bacilli made airborne by coughing; it is easily spread in crowded shelters or crowded apartments among those already in poor health. So housing as a problem is hardly unique to the AIDS population. But even if the housing problem is not distinctively an AIDS problem, many PWAs are homeless, and many are forced to spend time in the shelters, hardly an existence for terminally ill patients. Several respondents identified housing as the most serious problem for those diagnosed as having AIDS. From one to two thousand PWAs are estimated to have lost the battle for housing and to be seeking help in city shelters.

The most striking example of refusal to deal with a problem that is clearly within the mandate of the organization comes from an article by Dr. Don Des Jarlais, an expert on drugs and AIDS, and his co-workers, Cathy Casirel and Samuel Friedman. They describe the reactions of methadone-clinic workers—trained health workers who are presumably better equipped than the public at large to understand the AIDS problem —to the appearance of AIDS in the IVDU community and in their clinics. Their initial reaction to the possibility that there were AIDS carriers in the clinics was simply denial. They did not devote any resources to AIDS-related issues, they tried to screen out seropositive clients from the program, and they continued to treat their clients as if the epidemic would not affect them. The next stage was panic: they dismissed clients with AIDS when they learned of their seropositive status, or they required them to attend at difficult hours. In the third stage they finally cope, but there is a fourth stage, the authors tell us: burnout.[5]

We also heard many stories of nurses in hospitals who refused to have anything to do with AIDS patients because of the dangers of infection from casual contact. They are more highly trained than staff in methadone clinics. If trained health care workers such as these can refuse to have anything to do with AIDS, we should not be surprised at, for example, the strong resistance in workplaces even to using tools handled by persons with AIDS and the resistance to having children with AIDS in the schools.

Segregation and Inaction

Pattern D in Figure 8-1 indicates a means of dealing with AIDS by setting up task forces, coordinating units, special units, and the like—and delaying action. This response pattern may be considered

---

5. Des Jarlais, Casirel, and Friedman, "The New Death among IV Drug Users."

a natural second step once denial of the problem is no longer possible because the affected constituencies have gathered the necessary power to influence organizational policy. The combined use of patterns C and D is especially likely in the case of highly visible organizations that perceive blunt refusal or denial of the problem (pattern C) as politically damaging in the long run. Examples of this pattern would be expected to arise in the realm of public and government organizations at all levels, federal, state, county, and local.

The segregation strategy works as follows. A program that would normally have handled either PWAs or aspects of the AIDS problem —say, a health education program, an infectious disease unit, or the general office of the Social Security Administration—does not handle the AIDS problem or person as a matter of course, or perhaps even at all. Instead, one of two responses replaces direct action. First, a special AIDS unit such as a committee, coordinator, or office is set up to handle inquiries and plan for a response or to coordinate special actions by other newly formed units. A coordinating group may exist for months or years before anything is really done, as Shilts noted in his description of the task force within the New York City administration. The second response is creation of a segregated unit that does establish a program to provide care, research, or education, to process the disability claims, or whatever, but that is kept apart from the other programs.

Justifications are offered for both coordinating committees and special units, and sometimes the justifications are convincing. AIDS has unique characteristics and may deserve special treatment. Since it "covers the health map," as one respondent put it, and involves different diseases, social, financial, and legal problems, housing, prisons, employment problems, civil rights, and other issues, much coordination may be needed. But in our experience it was more often the case that the special unit or coordinating body was a device that prevented "contamination" of the normal tasks of the organization by AIDS and PWAs.

It is difficult to substantiate such a charge, because one cannot be sure about the motivations of others. For example, from our interviews we learned that the Social Security Administration office in New York managed to bar PWAs inquiring about or applying for their legal benefits from the reception room, on the grounds that their weakened immune systems put them at risk of picking up opportunistic infections from other visitors. An arrangement was made to handle applications and other matters by telephone; if a visit was necessary, the PWAs would go to a special office—to avoid exposure to all the diseases of the waiting room. (One may wonder which was the greater, fear for the health of the PWAs or fear for the health of others in the waiting room.) We suspect that the organization thought the mere presence of PWAs in a waiting room would affect its image. Disabled elderly persons could be accommodated without any stigma, but not PWAs. Fortunately, there was no evidence of delay or denial of service; indeed, the local Social Security Administration office appeared to have facilitated claims in several ways, thus helping PWAs. But for whatever reason, it managed to segregate the clients and the program from the rest of the organization.

Most organizations that are not concerned primarily with AIDS find that they have to establish a special task force or committee; the disease is different from most, and at the least a great deal of special education is required. But if AIDS presents the special kind of problem we have been asserting, we would expect coordination devices that minimize action and thus risks to take priority over direct service to the PWAs or groups at risk. It is not possible to prove this, but the extremely slow response of the New York State AIDS Institute, the ineffectual Office of Gay and Lesbian Health Concerns in New York City, criticisms we heard of some hospital responses, and even the extremely cautious, arm's-length way in which several organizations dealt with our requests for interviews through their public relations directors or AIDS coordinating unit directors, all point in that direction. These examples do not indicate outright refusals to deal with AIDS; but they do show that the problem was not welcomed into existing systems.

Distortion or Deflection of
Legitimate Organizational Goals

After segregation within the organization, the next most drastic consequence of the introduction of the AIDS problem to an organization is the distortion or deflection of the organization's legitimate purpose. We understood from an interview with a health educator at the New York City Department of Education that though AIDS education was a legitimate part of the health curriculum, and though that curriculum was given to the secondary schools, many schools refused to use it. The religious leaders on the school boards, Catholics in particular, objected. In fact, it was our understanding that the content of the curriculum was subject to unusual scrutiny and delay in the chancellor's office. If so, this would be a case of goal distortion; the health educational goals of the schools were subverted despite the recommendations of the Board of Education, and the educational program was modified as a result of unusual and perhaps unauthorized pressures. It would not surprise us if all this were true; the opposition of the Catholic Church to sex education even when the life of the student is at risk is well known. (After reading a draft of this section, however, our respondent denied that any of these problems had been mentioned in the interview. In the revised version of the respondent's story, the cooperation of the Catholic Church with the AIDS education efforts of the city's schools, for example, was described as excellent.)

An example of possible distortion or deflection concerns the dilemmas of the hospitals. By law hospitals cannot discharge an AIDS patient unless the patient has a suitable place to go—and homeless shelters are not considered suitable, for obvious reasons. But the hospitals are overcrowded; in the case of municipal hospitals, patients are being accommodated in emergency rooms for days or are kept in beds in the halls. They would be even more crowded if the increasing number of impoverished, homeless AIDS patients were to stay beyond the acute stage of their illness. (PWAs generally have two or three hospitalizations in the course of their disease, except for the very poor and isolated, who may have only a terminal admission.) We were told that doctors avoid giving a diagnosis of AIDS, so that the PWAs can be discharged to a homeless shelter or some other makeshift and exceedingly temporary arrangement, one consequence of which is that the statistics on the number of acute AIDS cases are distorted. Another consequence is that the health system does not have to own up to this particular failure. The most serious, of course, is the fate of ill patients.

A wider system effect can appear in this scenario. If the PWA goes to a shelter, as between one and two thousand were estimated to have done each night in 1988, they run the risk of being beaten up for having AIDS. Even worse, the shelters, just like the prisons, have instances of anal rape (and not necessarily by homosexual men). The PWA has the choice of warning the assailant of his condition, and probably being beaten up for having AIDS, or submitting and possibly passing on the deadly disease.[6] It is cases like this that seem to be without precedent in the history of epidemics among modern nations. Note the interaction of "failures": hospital overcrowding, deliberate misdiagnosis, homelessness, shelters that resemble prisons (but are better than the streets), the stigma and fear of AIDS, and the desperate sexual gratifications of social outcasts.

This pattern of distortion of organizational goals was illustrated in a December 1986 story in the *Wall Street Journal* about power and ideology in the Centers for Disease Control. (The story also touched on the next pattern, the disabling or destruction of a unit or its purpose.) Bureaucratic politics, jealousy, and conflict are to be expected even in organizations established to promote public welfare, but AIDS seems once again to have wreaked unusual havoc. The AIDS laboratory at the center was set up in 1983 and staffed with leading scientists. Yet of the six original senior scientists, five had left by the end of 1986, and of the five more who joined them in 1984, four were going, gone, or looking for other jobs. The lab had other unfilled positions and would have trouble staffing the new positions expected at the time the article was written.

Press reports led to a request by Senator Lowell Weicker of Connecticut for a study by the Institute of Medicine, part of the National Academy of Sciences. The institute reported, according to the *Wall Street Journal*, "that the AIDS lab has suffered from poor leadership, low morale, rivalries and distrust" and an atmosphere so bad that one scientist ordered the destruction of all the cultures, patiently nurtured, of

6. For an alarming but illuminating article on the homeless and PWAs, see Kolata, "New York Shelters, a Last Stop." No surveys that we were able to locate estimated the incidence of rape; staff members at the Coalition for the Homeless could only say that it exists, but they have no idea of the prevalence.

another scientist when he was out of town. Several other examples of mysteriously wrecked experiments are given. The issues at the lab involved (1) the competition between French and American scientists (Dr. Gallo was indirectly involved); (2) the authorship of papers (the director added his name as an author to papers with which he had almost no involvement); and (3) necessarily vague charges that the director of the lab was forced by pressures from the Reagan administration to delay or withhold support for a spermicide that killed the virus (thus presumably condoning nonmarital sex rather than abstinence). Scientists at the lab noted that a report by the Office of Technology Assessment on AIDS drew a conclusion that conformed to their own experience. One of the reasons, the report noted, that education efforts had received "minimal funding" by the administration was that "providing advice on preventive practices may be viewed as condoning bisexuality, homosexuality or intravenous drug abuse."[7] The CDC scientists felt that this criticism extended to their medical research.

As noted, these kinds of problems may occur in connection with research topics other than AIDS, but it would appear that they were especially severe in this case, severe enough to lead to the demoralization of those working on one of the key research weapons in the fight against AIDS. It is possible that this case is an exception, however. In another example of a federal program these kinds of problems were not experienced; indeed, in this case, AIDS produced a novel and creative response to a typical problem. It is worth examining briefly.

Four university labs and two pharmaceutical labs were funded to work on the AIDS virus in an attempt to find a way to block its destructive action. The unusual, perhaps unprecedented condition of the grants was that the four organizations had to meet together regularly and share one another's results prior to publication, in order to speed the research. We were told that the degree of cooperation varied "extremely," with some of the organizations living up to the requirement fully (including one of the for-profit pharmaceutical labs) and others hardly at all. But none of the issues that arose in the CDC case appeared.

7. Kwitny, "At CDC's AIDS Lab."

The problems of obtaining cooperation among the groups concerned the competition for the huge profits to be made on a drug that might affect several millions on a worldwide basis, and up to 1.5 million in the United States alone; for prestige in discovery; and for publications, especially for the graduate students and young professionals who could be hurt by the open-communication policy. Those problems would exist with research on other viruses, one assumes, so this is not a case of organizational failure because of AIDS. Indeed, we count this program as a success. It is striking, though, that such a novel contract would have to be written to speed AIDS research.

A second kind of goal deflection or distortion occurs when AIDS activates prejudices—anti-homosexual attitudes, racism, or personal fears—on the part of the organization's personnel or external constituencies. Organizations are places where many prejudices in society are expected to be held in check; organizations exist at the sufferance of society, because they draw upon so many of society's resources. In return, they are required to meet standards of behavior. However, organizations can find it difficult to maintain barriers against intolerant behavior; we suspect that AIDS had made it especially difficult to do so. It is clear that there is much anti-gay feeling, racism, and personal fearfulness of AIDS in the population, and grim stories of avoidance of PWAs and violation of their civil rights abound.[8] But it is even more disturbing when organizations cannot control these behaviors, because they are held to a higher standard than most individuals are. Yet there is evidence that school officials as well as parents have denied education rights to those who merely test positive for the antibodies, even though they are not a health threat. We were told several times of health care workers in hospitals who refused to carry out their duties with patients who had AIDS. The press has run stories of teachers, undertakers, dentists, surgeons, physicians, and other professionals who refuse to perform their professional tasks if AIDS is involved or even suspected. Police officers have gone to extreme lengths to protect themselves, in ways that suggest hostility to the stigmatized groups rather than professional behavior.

8. Conrad, "The Social Meaning of AIDS."

Although we have no concrete evidence, we expect that many of these reactions reflect racism as well as fear of contamination and homophobia. When the reactions occur in organizational settings, they do more than make it more difficult to achieve mandated goals; they oppose those goals and undo or reverse the established programs. In effect, they are sins of commission rather than omission.

Another example is the capitulation of the Roman Catholic Archdiocese of New York in 1985 to the petition of 400 parishioners opposing the location of a shelter for PWAs next door to a parochial school. This was the first concrete move of the archdiocese that we know of in the AIDS epidemic. The building was a former convent, and it already housed a women's shelter ("enough is enough," one irate parishioner said). The plan to use the shelter for PWAs was announced in a bulletin distributed at Sunday masses, by Wednesday the petition appeared, and on Thursday the plan was cancelled. While "saddened by the rejection," the pastor of the church added, "I can also understand the fear on the part of parents." Younger, more affluent families were moving into the neighborhood, the pastor noted, and this may have made it unsuitable for an AIDS shelter. Thus, the normal organizational response of defending the organization's programs against challenges, which in this case would have allowed the archdiocese to "reach out to those in need," as the disappointed pastor put it, was precluded by the specter of PWAs.[9]

Finally, there are organizations that are not mandated to provide services for PWAs or for the suffering, such as the National Hemophilia Foundation, but find that AIDS collides with their goals and weakens their ability to do their job. Hemophiliacs have been severely affected by AIDS. A blood-clotting product made of donated blood had increased their life span to near normal, but from about 1978 to 1985, until screening for AIDS in donated blood was finally in place, those requiring blood transfusions or the clotting product—most hemophiliacs—were at risk of infection. The rate of infection is assumed to be around 95 percent for the classic group of hemophiliacs ("Factor VIII hemophilia") and 65 percent for the rest. The disease is having a devastating effect

9. Sullivan, "Parishioners Block Archdiocese's AIDS Shelter."

upon the population: wives are divorcing husbands with AIDS; the disease has been transmitted to children; and a number of hemophiliacs have committed suicide. (Males have hemophilia; females carry the genes.)

The stigma attached to AIDS is penetrating; everything that comes into contact with the disease is affected. The impact extended to the National Hemophilia Foundation, which raises money for research and provides services for hemophiliacs and their families. The New York chapter experienced three problems: the recruitment of door-to-door fundraisers fell off, prestigious members began to leave the board of directors, and two foundations that had provided the bulk of the funding withdrew their support. Why? For the fundraisers and the volunteer board members, it was the association with AIDS and all that AIDS is associated with. Hemophiliacs were dying of AIDS, a disease of gay men and minorities. They looked for less controversial places to give their volunteer services. For the foundations, it was a matter of triage: the hemophilia population was largely doomed anyway, so they decided their funds should go elsewhere. (This is the argument that is sometime whispered in New York City regarding expensive care for dying PWAs, as if the dying have lost their rights to succor and compassion.) Fortunately, the National Hemophilia Foundation has managed to raise funds from several other sources.

AIDS Disables or Destroys the Organization

Pattern F in Figure 8-1 suggests that AIDS can be as destructive of programs and normal responsibilities as it is of the human body. In some cases an ongoing program or an accepted responsibility is disabled or destroyed when AIDS enters the picture. Denial, segregation, or goal distortion will not work as a defense in these cases. The example of the CDC lab reported above is illustrative of how AIDS may eventually destroy the basic parameters along which organized work proceeds. In another example, reported to us by the head of a community agency but not otherwise verified by us, a Brooklyn hospital had an elite medical team that dealt with unusual or very difficult cases. Its record was excellent and morale was high. It seemed logical for the team to take responsibility for AIDS cases, so it got all the referrals. Within a few months the special team had to be abandoned. Morale had dropped, burnout was reported for the first time, turnover, which had been very low, zoomed, and infighting over the technical and ethical problems involved in AIDS took its toll. What these two cases suggest is that organizational units that are small, self-contained, and clearly focused might be severely impaired and even destroyed if they fail to deal with AIDS as successfully as they have dealt with other problems.

Families and communities appear to be as vulnerable as organizations. A revealing though nonorganizational example concerns reports of families in the Hispanic community refusing to take in and care for family members with AIDS. We are sure that this occurs in all groups of our society, but it was more striking here because of the high value placed on family life and care in Hispanic culture. A social worker reported that she might have to work for two or three weeks to get all family members to agree to take back a family member about to be discharged from the hospital with an AIDS diagnosis. The alternatives were bleak—either a false diagnosis so that the patient could be sent to a homeless shelter or a brief stop at some makeshift arrangement and then on to the streets. For the family, it would appear that the "shame" of homosexuality, bisexuality, or intravenous drug use was sometimes too great.

SUMMARY

This litany of organizational failures is not meant to be exhaustive, and individual cases could be analyzed in more than one way. These are the kinds of obstacles organizations will confront when coping with unusual degrees of stigma, fear, and expense. Neither our current conservative ideology, our health sector, nor our slums provide a context that encourages organizations to overcome obstacles and at least adhere to expected standards of behavior. Any disease or other social problem will present challenges to existing organizations, and organizations are always falling short. But AIDS presents unique and unusually fierce problems. It is striking to find the New York chapter of the Hemophiliac

Foundation colliding with images of gay men and IVDUs in its attempts to provide service to hemophiliacs and their families. One does not expect research labs at the Centers for Disease Control to have experiments destroyed and questions raised about the morality of sexual behavior in connection with its work. And it is surprising to find that almost no existing organizations with mandates in the health or housing areas have incorporated, without resistance, PWAs with health and housing problems.

We think it is useful to conceive of organizations as in considerable part concerned with preventing denial, flight, goal distortion, and discrimination in connection with their public charge. (All organizations, even private ones, have public charges and are subject to laws and lawsuits, to scrutiny of their behavior to a degree, and to an implicit understanding that they exist by the consent of the society.) Organizational failure is a more serious matter than, say, the inefficient use of human and societal resources or the use of faulty strategies, especially when crises arise. Organizations draw on societal resources and have subtle powers to shape our lives; we have a right to expect them to be responsive to emergencies such as the AIDS epidemic. Indeed, since large organizations have, so to speak, absorbed so much of what we once thought of as society, since they shape our lives so pervasively from conception to death, it is inconceivable that a serious social problem such as an epidemic could have any other solution or mitigation than an organizational one.[10] AIDS is as much an organizational problem as a biological one; we have long since passed the point where individual behavior alone could be held responsible for the epidemic or for its amelioration and termination. AIDS in the United States was borne and spread by organizations in a very real sense; individuals die from it

10. The "absorption of society by organizations" is a theme of Charles Perrow's paper, "A Society of Organizations," Yale University, 1989. It predicts that as small, flexible, and locally responsive organizations disappear into large public and private bureaucracies, the possibility of the unexpected interaction of failures among these large, inflexible organizations increases, and the buffer of small organizations disappears and cannot be replaced in time. The result is "system accidents." This has been the implicit theme of our analysis of AIDS.

because of organizations; organizations will provide whatever succor and dignity will attend those deaths; and the dying will stop because of organizations. But, as we have seen, the defenses of organizations are weak in the face of the stigma, fears, and costs of AIDS. Organizations can spread AIDS, but as recalcitrant tools in the service of diverse interest groups, they have performed very poorly in coping with it.

9   AIDS UNENDING

Only three things could stop AIDS from becoming the epidemic of the century in the United States and the world: a new disease
even more widely spread, control of the infections the virus unleashes,
or development of a vaccine within a very few years. It is already the
epidemic of the second half of the century. A new disease is not out of
the question; it is possible that AIDS was present in Africa for some
decades and required only an effective way to get from isolated groups
into the jetstream of world travel. Control, or a way of holding the
diseases associated with HIV at bay, is very likely and may have happened already. As of this writing, the drug AZT is thought to be capable
of suppressing symptoms among those who are HIV-positive; if that is
true AIDS may be treated as a chronic disease that can be controlled,
very much like diabetes. (The virus changes to tolerate AZT, however,
so a range of similar drugs is needed.) A tested, approved vaccine seems
to be several years off.

Barring these developments, the disease is likely to surpass the
influenza epidemic of 1918–1919 before the turn of the century in the
number of deaths it causes. We have vastly more resources today than
were available at the time of that epidemic for understanding and caring
for people struck by an epidemic and for educating others about prevention. Unlike any other epidemic we know of, AIDS can be prevented at a
cost, in the United States, of only a couple of dollars spent in a super-

market or drugstore. Unlike any other, it has been visited overwhelmingly on stigmatized groups in our society (though not everywhere in the world). We have argued that the stigma attached to the groups most heavily affected has made an effective response very difficult for the variety of health, educational, and political organizations that should have dealt with the epidemic. Also important was the fear the disease generates—the fear of unknown transmission, of transmission by casual contact, of long latency periods, and so on. And, finally, we feel that many organizations did not respond appropriately because of the sheer cost that could be expected, perhaps in the hope that the next level of government would step in and pay.

Most existing organizations that had a mandate to deal with the problem failed grievously, we believe. Some did not, and some recovered after initial failures, but organizations in both categories are in the minority. We have tried to detail and explain the failure. But beyond this level of inadequate action on the part of specific organizations—such as blood banks, hospitals, churches, and housing departments (and many others that we have not mentioned, such as insurance companies, drug companies, police departments, business and industrial organizations that have discriminated)—is a larger failure. It appears to us that we citizens of the United States simply have not cared enough, if at all, about the suffering and the death of thousands of our fellow citizens. How are we to explain not only the failure of our organizations but the failure of our society as well?

In this book we have emphasized the two major groups of persons with AIDS. Gays still account for the bulk of the cases, but cases among IVDUs are increasing fast. Yet a third group, women partners of IVDUs and their children, is growing at an alarming rate. A fourth group, those infected via heterosexual transmission, now largely associated with crack use, is also rising. This is the method whereby the heterosexual population in the United States is, at present, most likely to be infected. (In Africa it is overwhelmingly a heterosexual population that is affected.)

Figure 9-1 outlines the dynamics of the spread of AIDS in the United States since the 1970s. It shows the progression of the disease as recognized by health officials; it does not indicate the actual progression, of

Figure 9-1. *Paths of HIV transmission in the United States of dominant concern since the 1970s*

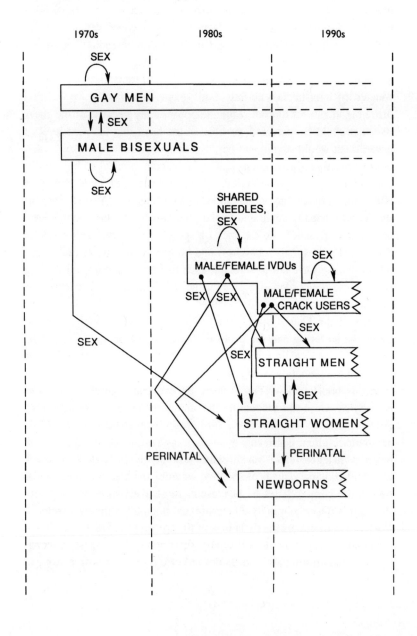

which we know little. Nor does it reflect the number of infected people in the categories or the transmission of AIDS through the donation of blood. Initially, gay men and bisexuals infected each other, and IVDUs (males and females, but mostly males) infected each other. The disease was more or less "dead-ended" with these two groups, with some extension to the sexual partners of bisexuals and especially of the IVDUs and to the children of these female partners. But this extension to women was not a well-traveled route, nor one that then extended to non-drug-using males. The sexual partners of male IVDUs were probably more likely to have sex with other infected IVDUs than with non-drug-using heterosexuals, though this is just a guess.

With the introduction of crack smoking and the sexual behaviors associated with it, the population at risk of AIDS expanded. Some of those participating in crack-smoking bouts were seropositive IVDUs. Through repeated and prolonged sexual activity, they infected female crack smokers. Non-IVDUs, males and females, also participated in these crack-smoking activities, becoming infected as a result. They, in turn, could have sexual partners who were non-drug-using heterosexuals. In this way, the virus has the potential for breaking out of the IVDU group and even the crack-smoking group, but as of this writing there was no evidence of a surge of cases among non-drug-using heterosexuals. The children of infected women were estimated to have a 50 percent chance of being HIV-positive.

Gays were the easiest "test" of our society's sincerity: they were overwhelmingly white, many were very accomplished and well connected, and because of their career successes and life-style (often two incomes with no children) they were more affluent than the average family. In San Francisco they also had considerable political power. And they took steps—late, we think, but eventually—to reduce the risks of transmission. Yet the federal government was deplorably slow to act, as virtually every one of the prestigious reports and studies agreed, discrimination increased, and in New York State and City the response was as tardy and as ineffectual as at the national level. Now the inevitable progress of the epidemic will continue to kill thousands of gays each year for the next decade or so. Only medication to control the infection or an outright cure will stop what Shilts has called the "avalanche of deaths." And while the disease is no longer spreading at an epidemic rate in the gay community, as far as can be determined, new cases (boys), continued institutional sources of infection (commercial establishments such as cinemas), male prostitution, and the inevitable risks taken in some sexual encounters leave a great deal to be done in education and prevention.

Looking back over the "sexual revolution," "gay pride," "gay liberation," and "coming out of the closet," we believe that the virus in the United States interacted fatally with a brief but dramatic episode in the history of homosexual behavior. The distinguishing features of this episode—the gay clubs and bathhouses and the macho, aggressive culture of a segment of the gay community in the 1970s and the 1980s—were ideally suited to dissemination of the virus. It seems reasonable to assume that if antihomosexual attitudes in society, attitudes tied to our religious fundamentalism and fear of rapid social changes, were not present, the assertive cultural expression of the gay sexual revolution would not have been so widespread. (We have no evidence for this of course, nor could we have.) Frequent, anonymous sex in an aggressive form could still have occurred, and indeed is still celebrated as right by some,[1] but would not have been so prevalent. Instead, men could have lived together openly in far more stable relationships. Discrimination against homosexuality promoted the kinds of behavior that most of us would call extreme on

---

1. For example, Martin Duberman, a prominent historian, decries the purported increased acceptance of homosexuals by heterosexuals on the basis of reductions in flamboyant sexual behavior. Duberman sees the sexual conduct that has been curtailed not as a product of the discrimination gays have experienced but as something to be valued. Nor is it a mistake, to be given up because of medical necessity. He is quoted in the press as saying, "The cost [of acceptance by heterosexuals] could be our soul and part of our heritage. I read that our community has 'matured' and I want to vomit. Under the leash of necessity we have curtailed our sexual conduct. But it is quite another thing to reread our history and declare it a mistake" Gross, "Amid Bias, Homosexuals Are Finding New Understanding.") Some gay spokespersons, perhaps most, still argue that the bathhouses should not have been closed. See the article by Mark S. Senak, director of legal services at the Gay Men's Health Crisis, in *AIDS and the Law* (Senak, "The Lesbian and Gay Community," pp. 293–294).

the part of what surely was a relatively small minority of gays. It was a large enough minority to sustain an epidemic that could spread to those not caught up in the culture of multiple partners.

Even without the fear of AIDS we believe that the behaviors of male homosexuals that seem so extreme to straight society would have moderated a great deal. Given the stigma and the discrimination attached to gay behavior, it would have been difficult for some to avoid those extremes. But, we hasten to say, we are not experts on this subject, have no data on it, and hold these views very tentatively. We believe the matter should be explored by those who know more than we do. In any case, the most dangerous practices have diminished greatly (though they have not disappeared) in just a few years, if we can accept the evidence of a few surveys (but not all) and especially of the decline in the rate of increase of HIV-positive gay and bisexual males.

With regard to IVDUs, it seems clear that society does not care. Some people obviously do, including those who work in the field of drug rehabilitation, but in general IVDUs are even more victimized than gay men are. They were hardly noticed until the mid 1980s and still appear to receive far less governmental and voluntary assistance than is available to gay men. And yet society as a whole is heavily implicated in the creation of the drug market that the IVDU population is caught up in.

The connection between middle-class substance abuse (including alcoholism and tranquilizing drugs) and substance abuse in the lower class is intimate. But while there are at least some services and some little tolerance for middle-class drug abuses, there is none for the lower class. Drug abuse can be motivated by the search for exquisite pleasures and thrills and by peer-group norms. Perhaps a good part of middle-class abuse is of this sort. But if drug abuse can also result from avoidance behavior, if people are driven to it out of desperation about their human condition, it is all the more understandable in the slums and ghettos of our cities than in the high-rise apartments and the greening suburbs. Furthermore, if there were not a large market for illegal drugs among the nonpoor, the poor would not be dealing in drugs as much as they are and using the profits to experiment and get addicted themselves. The following scenario, although it is obviously oversimplified, will serve to make our point about blaming and thus rejecting those who are the real victims of the majority's vulnerability to drugs.

Rich and middle-class kids abuse drugs for thrills, pleasures, and peer acceptance. The demand creates an illegal market for drugs. It is most practically serviced by poor kids, who live where police surveillance is low and the dealers have little to lose if caught. The business is very profitable because of the risk; many profit and few get caught. With illicit cash in their pockets and drugs passing through their hands, more poor kids are vulnerable to using drugs than the rich kids. The poor kids start tasting their wares and become addicted. Addiction grows, so profits must grow, but the middle- and upper-class market may not expand enough to support the new expensive habits. Therefore the poor who are dealing in drugs have to sell to their neighbors in order to expand their sales and pay for their habit. Their neighbors are poor, so it is hard to afford a habit. But since the neighbors are poor they are vulnerable to addiction. Like the pushers, they are easy to recruit into aggressive marketing or pushing in their own community. They may have to commit crimes against their own neighbors to support their habit, creating more social dislocation than can be ameliorated by drugs.

Demand declines among the rich kids who started it all because they are not in desperate circumstances and thus are less vulnerable. But it rises among the poor. The rate of increase will vary with the degree to which the drug is addictive and its cost. The higher the addictiveness and the lower the cost, the more rapid the spread. Crack is addictive and cheap. If crack can spread viruses as well as addictions, the problems of disease and drug abuse are compounded, for the social upheaval created by many people walking around with deadly viruses and dying from them increases the desperation that can feed drug habits. Drugs and AIDS are negatively synergistic in ways in which homosexual behavior and AIDS are not. The drug component of the AIDS epidemic is thus potentially more catastrophic.

Another negative synergy associated with drugs is worth mentioning; it too indicates middle- and upper-class complicity in catastrophic events. The cocaine problem in the 1980s is a classic instance of negative synergy on a worldwide basis. Recent news stories have outlined a chain of events that links air pollution in pristine parts of our continent and world to the enormous demand for cocaine in the United States, an unknown but significant proportion of which must come from the middle and upper classes. Because of the demand for cocaine and the illegality of the drug, gigantic profits can be made by supplying the cocaine. Peru, a desperately poor country, has an ideal environment for growing coca plants, high in the Andes. To grow them, the fragile mountain soil must be stripped of its vegetation with toxic defoliants, planted with coca plants, and fertilized with strong chemicals. The defoliants, fertilizers, and, later, the processing chemicals flow into the headwaters of the Amazon, polluting it and killing the fish.

Because of poverty in the country and its particular political circumstances, an extremist "Maoist" revolutionary group, the Shining Path, flourishes. The Shining Path protects the drug lords from government attempts to wipe out their growing and refining operations. (These are local drug lords; the main ones are headquartered in Colombia, where the final processing and distribution take place.)

But more important than the pollution of the rivers and the erosion of the soil as it is quickly exhausted by the coca plants, the rain forests that are thought to help cleanse the atmosphere of the industrialized nations' pollutants are rapidly being destroyed. Their destruction is hastened so that the demand for cocaine in North America can be satisfied.

Obviously, our cities are being damaged by drug addiction and the drug trade. To the apparent costs of addiction we can add the fouling of the very air, something that the rich and poor of all nations depend upon. This is not a chain of events the United States can be proud of. The failures of organizations that we have been describing are overwhelmed by the more massive failure of social structure (responsible for the poverty that encourages addiction and trafficking) and culture (a repugnance toward abusers that forestalls an admission of compliance and thus makes prevention and rehabilitation efforts trivial).

INEQUALITY IN AMERICA

The failure of social structure and culture is not inevitable; European democracies do better than we do—some, as in Scandinavia, far better. (As crack invades Europe that may change, but the more "benign" phases of the AIDS epidemic have been handled better elsewhere.) Our poor record has a lot to do with our culture of racism, which has less of a role in Europe. But it seems to us that the new locus of infectivity, in the minority and drug-using population, is a result of fairly recent failures in our society that have increased poverty and drug abuse. To examine these, we must back up a bit.

The United States in the first half of the nineteenth century was a surprisingly egalitarian society by today's standards. Inequality of wealth and income rose steadily with industrialization, which concentrated wealth and income.[2] By the end of the century a reaction had set in. Labor unions and social movements bloomed, disappeared for a time with a series of depressions and panics, and reemerged in the early twentieth century. From about 1870 to 1970 it took a series of political efforts and even some fierce social movements to prevent the increase in the inequality of wealth and income, which presumably was the inevitable tendency of capitalism. The expanding franchise, a court system that finally began to redress the imbalance of power between employers and employees to some extent, radical unions and the "progressive movement" early in the twentieth century, the beginnings of a welfare state in the Great Depression, resurgent labor shortly afterward, the civil rights movement of 1950s and 1960s, and various liberation movements in the 1960s—all these just managed to keep the level of inequality from increasing. Inequality in the United States has been among the highest in industrialized nations.

Inequality increased gradually in the 1970s and sharply in the 1980s. First, the United States lost its economic and political hegemony in the world. We produced about three-quarters of the gross world output at the end of World War II and less than one-quarter by 1980. There was bound to be a large change, but in the 1950s and 1960s we were able to

2. Williamson and Lindert, *American Inequality*.

dominate the world politically and economically and to enjoy unparalleled prosperity. Blacks, the only significant minority then in terms of numbers, were being integrated into the industrial economy and the cities, and it appeared that things could only get better for them. Poverty was declining steadily. The last major impoverished group, the aged, were making steady gains and eventually were above average in income (as the income of children fell). As agriculture became mechanized in the South, industry in the North absorbed the emigrating black population.

Around 1965 signs appeared that we had serious economic competitors in Germany and Japan, and by 1973 it was clear that political resurgence among the Moslem countries meant that we no longer had political hegemony. Accustomed to dominance abroad, the American public was shocked by oil cartels, terrorism, hostages, and the continuing Arab-Israeli wars. At home, manufacturing jobs were disappearing and imports rising. Social programs picked up some of the slack in the economy caused by declining cities and unemployment and inflation. But after the 1980 election social programs as remedies were curtailed, and a new administration, promising a resurgence of political, military, and economic dominance in the world, turned aside from social problems. A sharp recession was produced, increasing the poverty rate and reducing the power and membership of unions. Then social programs were cut. Housing programs were cut (and, as we have recently seen, corrupted), and the homeless appeared; prenatal and infant health programs were cut, and infant mortality rates rose along with premature births and associated disabilities and retardation; unions were attacked, and the relative level of wages stagnated and then fell; tax cuts grossly favored the rich, and the average family's inflation-adjusted income fell; the class structure elongated, as the standard of living for the poorest fifth of the population fell by 9 percent between 1979 and 1987 while the living standard of the highest fifth rose by 19 percent. The credo of the decade was to "get government off our backs"; with decreased regulation, the infrastructure of the cities decayed, the environment got worse, and fraud and economic concentration in deregulated industries such as transportation and banking increased. Meanwhile, our public debt soared, and so did the trade imbalance. Our political and economic decline in the world became the subject of daily headlines.[3]

It is in this context—one of political ideology exploiting public fears —that we must see the appearance of AIDS and our response to it. With a deteriorating health sector and rapidly deteriorating cities and ghettos within them, a disease that found a place to live and prosper among the poor was bound to spread. The section on the minority community in Chapter 6 gives some indication of conditions there and of the rapid changes in the black population in the past two decades. It suggests the irrelevancy of most of the responses made by existing organizations and even by the new ones struggling to deal with AIDS.

Here we would like to highlight the picture of poverty in New York City in order to illustrate more clearly, and once again, a major theme of our work: the interrelatedness of the problems, or the negative synergy revealed by a systems analysis. We will present a list of brief "takes" largely from the *New York Times* at the close of the 1980s. The decay of the city is too recent to be reflected in scholarly works; even William Wilson's book *The Truly Disadvantaged*, had to a large extent draw upon surveys and studies from the 1970s as it focused on the problems of the 1980s.

HOSPITALS AND CLINICS

The number of advisory panels and commissioned reports concerned with the hospital and health care crisis continues to grow. The March 1989 report of a mayoral panel, established the previous September, was typical in its very strong language and dire warnings. AIDS, it said, "threatens to become the city's social catastrophe of this century." It is the final straw "which threatens the well-being of the entire system and the availability of health care for all New Yorkers." Without action, the panel warned, "the whole proud New York City system of

3. Bowles, Gordon, and Weisskopf, *Beyond the Wasteland*; Harrison and Bluestone, *The Great U-Turn*; Thurow, "A Surge in Inequality"; Wilson, *The Truly Disadvantaged*; and Perrow, "A Society of Organizations."

patient care, biomedical research and medical training, generally viewed as the best in the world, will swiftly deteriorate."[4] (Note the emphasis on the consequences for reputations and the nonpoor.) New York City is not alone. A report in the *Journal of the American Medical Association* detailed the problem for the nation as a whole. The greatest rate of growth in AIDS cases is in the South and Midwest, but meanwhile, 20 percent of the hospitals, most in a few large urban areas, provided 77 percent of the care in 1987. The average public hospital in New England and the South lost over $600,000 on AIDS cases that year, because of the low level of reimbursement.[5] This figure does not reflect the General Accounting Office estimate that only two-thirds of AIDS and other fatal HIV-related illnesses are captured in official forecasts.[6] As of November 1989, 12,803 persons had officially died of AIDS in New York City, but, according to one news report that year citing "city researchers," about 2,500 others have died of the disease without ever having been treated or even diagnosed; presumably most died in hospitals with other diagnoses. Public and private hospitals in the city housed an average of 1,800 AIDS patients a day, but we do not know how many other patients were not officially diagnosed as such; $700 million from all sources that year was being spent on AIDS from all sources in the city.[7] The city cut the Health and Hospitals Corporation and Health Department budgets in 1987, restored the cuts and added a little more money in 1988, but "a widely respected vice president of the agency," according to a *New York Times* reporter, quit the HHC in protest over the inadequate budget, and the head of the flagship Bellevue Hospital Center was fired after refusing to make cuts that she said imperiled patient care.[8]

4. Lambert, "AIDS Patients Seen Straining Hospitals."
5. Lambert, "Concentration of AIDS Cases"; Andrulis, Weslowski, and Gage, "The 1987 U.S. Hospital AIDS Survey."
6. "Forecasts of AIDS Fall Short." See also Laumann et al., "Monitoring the AIDS Epidemic in the United States."
7. Lambert: "AIDS Services: A Disjointed Network." See also Siegel, "The Wall-to-Wall Emergency at City Hospitals," for a graphic description of the crowding and tension. Such accounts are frequent in the *New York Times*.
8. Lambert, "Debate Swirls over Cuts."

New York is not the only city in trouble, of course, just the biggest. In Oakland, California, across the bay from San Francisco, a reporter notes that crack "has turned emergency medicine at Highland General Hospital here into a nightmare, a scene of chaos and despair that is crushing the spirits of all who encounter it." In the worst areas of Oakland, Los Angeles, and New York, half the emergency-room patients are drug users. They are abusive, fight off staff and police, frequently require restraints, beat up psychiatrists doing interviews, and return time and again for wounds, overdoses, psychotic episodes, or exposure. On the rare occasion that one seeks help in overcoming the addiction, all that can be done is to put him or her on the waiting list for treatment, some months off. In a twelve-hour survey of all admissions on a Saturday night in the Oakland hospital, every urine sample tested positive for cocaine. The staff are all trained in self-defense, and interviews are held in halls, where police are stationed. (Involuntary medication to quell violent behavior is illegal.) Some patients arrive with thousands of dollars in their pockets. When challenged about his career choice, a teenaged bookkeeper in a crack house said, "I'm not going to work for chump change. I make $2,000 a week, tax free. What do they pay you, sucker?" Not nearly that much, concluded the physician. Crack-related admissions peak after welfare checks arrive. Ambulance paramedics answered an emergency call about a premature delivery of an infant and found the mother smoking a crack pipe while waiting. Crack families "triage themselves," casting out the most unruly and thieving of their members. A doctor reported: "Sometimes I call and they say 'Keep the boy,' and hang up the phone."[9]

Gunshot wounds, related in large part to drug wars, cost this hospital $10.5 million in two years—700 victims. Because many are caused by assault rifles, which are still made in the United States (Congress and the President have refused to ban them), heroic surgical procedures are required. It was estimated by a study reported in the *Journal of the American Medical Association* that the cost of treating gun wounds nationwide was $1 billion annually. "Trench medicine," the head of the

9. Gross, "Emergency Room: A Crack Nightmare."

emergency room called their work; the director of trauma services at a Los Angeles hospital said, "These are war injuries, period, end of discussion."[10] They are certainly not hunting accidents. These are the mean streets of our social policy, into which AIDS slips as just another way to die.

The Oakland hospital may be lucky that it is not being closed. Interfaith hospital in central Brooklyn runs out of basic supplies repeatedly, and doctors pitch in to buy sutures and equipment; the hospital owed $16 million to its suppliers in March 1989, and the state threatened to close it because of hospital-code violations. But it is the community's only source of health care (and ironically, as a symbol of our inner-city social policy, its largest employer); it serves a half-million citizens in an area with some of the highest rates of infant mortality, drug use, violence, and, of course, AIDS in New York City. It is under constant threat of closure because of debts and code violations.[11] When we visited the harried AIDS staff in 1987 we found jammed halls, cramped, poorly lighted rooms, wards crammed with beds, and a remarkable staff hanging on somehow in the face of desperate and occasionally aggressive patients.

All hospitals are affected by the crisis; voluntary (private, nonprofit) hospitals are required to provide care for the poor, and while some are able to keep Medicaid admissions down to as little as 2.3 percent, the average was 22.4 percent for 1987. This has spawned complaints of the "municipalization" of voluntary hospitals, which are swamped with Medicaid admissions, for which only three-quarters or so of the cost of care is covered, and with the growing number of citizens who lack even this much protection, for whom reimbursement from the city may be as low as 10 percent. In 1988 two voluntary hospitals had to close their outpatient pharmacies, which provided subsidized medicine for the poor. One was Mount Sinai Medical Center in Manhattan. The other was Columbia Presbyterian, in upper Manhattan near Columbia University. It has a

10. Gross, "Epidemic in Urban Hospitals."
11. Howard W. French, "In Brooklyn, a Hospital Faces Its Own Mortality," *New York Times*, March 20, 1989.

clientele of middle-class patients but also serves a sizable poor population. Its pharmacy was said to be one of the most receptive to the poor, but the hospital is reimbursed only 10 cents on the dollar for uninsured patients. In the past ten years *five* of the hospitals above 140th Street in Manhattan have closed. This is Harlem. Because of the nursing shortage Columbia cannot open 200 new beds in one building. In five years of a mounting health crisis in the city, Columbia-Presbyterian has been forced to make three layoffs, the most recent of 300 personnel.[12] In Oakland, California, the only clinic providing routine health care to the bulk of the city's poor closed in February 1989 because of insufficient reimbursement of medical costs, which have risen dramatically because of the crack epidemic. It served nearly 9,000 recipients of the state's medical insurance program for the poor.[13]

HOMELESSNESS

AIDS interacts with other social problems, as we have said repeatedly. The homeless problem has a very prosaic source: mental patients were turned out into the streets; more important, funds for subsidized housing for the poor were cut, even while financial benefits were available for housing for the well-to-do; in New York City developers of commercial office space and expensive condominiums benefitted from handsome tax breaks. City leaders and the mass media celebrated the life-styles of conspicuous consumers such as Donald Trump. Nationally, funding for housing under the Department of Housing and Urban Development (HUD) fell by two-thirds between 1981 and 1986, the largest cut for a cabinet-level department in the Reagan Administration, and HUD-subsidized housing starts went from 144,348 to only 17,080 units (and much of even this small effort benefitted ineligible people because of corrupt administration). Meanwhile subsidies in the form of tax deductions for mortgages, which greatly favor those at the upper income lev-

---

12. French, "Again, Debate Over Private Hospitals' Public Duty"; Lyall, "Hospital Calls Layoff of 300 a Last Resort."
13. Bishop, "Gap between Cost of Drug Epidemic and State Money."

els, totaled $42.4 billion in 1986, when all HUD housing programs were only $10 billion.[14] (The scandals of mismanagement during the Reagan years, disclosed in 1989, may, according to an early estimate, have cost as much as $2 billion.)[15]

The homeless situation, a result of deliberate policies with quite predictable outcomes, so outraged ten of the thirteen members of a National Academy of Sciences (NAS) panel of experts asked to make a study of it that they took the virtually unprecedented step of privately publishing an addendum to the official report. The addendum, using language the Academy would not permit in its version, described homelessness in the United States as "an outrage, a national scandal." These experts also objected to the limited nature of the recommendations permitted in the official report, arguing that they failed to address the problem.

The National Academy had refused to publish the supplementary statement because the language was too charged. The president of the Academy, Dr. Frank Press, acknowledged that the panel members were repelled by what they had found but argued that they still could not go beyond the fact-finding report that had been requested and give their own views. (The three panel members who agreed with Dr. Press and refused to sign the supplementary statement were, perhaps characteristically, an academic economist, a medical school dean, and the head of a Washington-based consulting firm.) The Academy was practicing its own form of "just saying no" in the face of a national scandal; otherwise it might lose its credibility. The "intrusion of values," Dr. Press was quoted as saying, "must be minimized as much as possible" in Academy reports.[16]

Estimates of the number of homeless vary greatly. The NAS report used those of a 1988 study, which found 735,000 Americans homeless on any given night, with 1.3 to 2 million homeless for one night or more during the year. The supplementary statement found this to be "an inexcusable disgrace [which] must be eliminated." Here is a sample of the

14. Swanstrom, "Homeless: A Product of Policy."
15. Johnston, "Radical Rehab."
16. Boffey, "Homeless Plight Angers Scientists."

passion that Dr. Press, the Academy, and three of the panel members found inappropriate:

> We can no longer sit as spectators to the elderly homeless dying of hypothermia, to the children with blighted futures poisoned by lead in rat-infested dilapidated welfare hotels, to women raped, to old men beaten and robbed of their few possessions, and to people dying on the streets with catastrophic illnesses such as AIDS.[17]

Attempts to solve an obvious problem in New York City and in the nation have been, at best, lacking in vigor. Congress passed the requisite bill in 1987 to force the federal government to make unused or underused federal properties available for the homeless, but almost nothing happened. An advocacy group, the National Coalition for the Homeless, brought suit against the government for violating the new law, and the federal district judge agreed. Only twelve facilities out of tens of thousands of potential ones were identified by federal agencies, and only two were made available to the homeless a year later.[18] Similarly glacial movement characterizes the situation in New York City. Eight years into the epidemic the city has only one small site devoted to homeless AIDS patients, numbering an estimated 1,000–2,000; it is Bailey House, in the West Village. Three residential AIDS centers were to be built in 1987, but the (quite predictable) local opposition and the expense involved defeated two of them. In October 1988, plans for eight sites in three boroughs were announced. The opposition of two of the three borough presidents was swift, predictable, and may be decisive. (David Dinkins, then Manhattan Borough President, was not opposed, though four of the eight sites were in his borough.) The two opponents claimed they had not been consulted, but Mayor Koch claimed that they had been asked for recommendations but had given none.[19] One might be forgiven for suspecting that all are correct, that the mayor was aware that

17. Quoted in Boffey, "Homeless Plight Angers Scientists."
18. "Administration Faulted on Homeless Aid Program."
19. Marriott, "Koch Picks 8 Sites in 3 Boroughs"; Homeless AIDS Patients"; McFadden, "Koch Criticized on Plan."

the borough presidents would blame the lack of consultation and that the matter will be stalled while all save face. If a shelter is begun, the local community can stall or halt its completion, as they have done with drug-counseling centers such as ADAPT and methadone clinics. Attacks on homosexuals in the United States are increasing, according to the National Gay and Lesbian Task Force, with 625 reported in New York state in 1988, so homeless shelters for AIDS patients are doubly controversial.[20]

Neither Koch, no longer the mayor, nor the borough presidents can be expected to suffer for their inaction, though the long-run costs for the communities will be heavy. As the homeless population gets larger, its members experiencing more permanent rather than transitory bouts of homelessness, street tensions will rise, the attitudes of those with homes will harden against those without them, and a sense of community will decline. Harassment of those with homes increases as the long-term homeless get more aggressive. And presumably this kind of deterioration of a neighborhood leads to increased drug addiction and crime. It becomes harder and harder for people to care.

CHILDREN

The major cause of death in poor children used to be infectious diseases. The death rate has increased recently; however, the major causes are no longer infections but the blame-shifting term "diseases of lifestyle," which, according to Mayor Koch's panel, might better be called "diseases of despair"—pediatric AIDS, child abuse, and substance abuse. They threaten the future of a generation of children, the report said, and the city has responded "inadequately." Of the 2 million children in New York City, almost 25 percent have no health insurance, and about 60 percent are living in poor or near-poor families. The report, two years in the making, was finished in May 1989 but was not made public until it was leaked to the press in late July of that year, amid charges that Mayor Koch did not like its findings and so delayed releasing it. Its recommendations are as mild as its indictment of the city and

20. Gutis, "Attacks on U.S. Homosexuals Held Alarmingly Widespread."

state government—for example, to raise to only 50 percent the percentage of pregnant substance-abusing women enrolled in drug-treatment programs.[21]

As AIDS interacts with poverty and drug abuse, it generates new tragedies. First, women who were sexual partners of IVDUs became infected. Then their children. And now, inexorably, AIDS has spawned a generation of orphans—children who are not themselves, infected but who have lost their parents to the disease. On the Lower East Side of Manhattan a support group has been formed for primary school children whose parents are dying or have died of AIDS. Bruce Lambert, in one of several remarkable articles he wrote on the disease, remarked on an eight-year-old boy who had brought a photo of his father lying dead in his coffin to the session: "This is show-and-tell in the age of AIDS."

A City Health Department doctor estimates that by 1995 there will be 20,000 orphans of AIDS needing adoption or foster care. The agencies charged with caring for orphans will be overloaded—just one more example, after the failures in housing, nursing homes, hospital beds, nursing supply, drug clinics, and so on, of AIDS defeating an impoverished and floundering service.[22] And more and more families will be shouldering an all-but-impossible responsibility, like the one described in Lambert's article: "A Manhattan woman with seven adult children has lost three to AIDS, and the fourth is dying. She and an uninfected daughter are now trying to care for 10 orphaned grandchildren."[23]

DRUGS AND CRACK

We have portrayed AIDS as unique among epidemics because of the stigma and fear attached to the disease and the cost of fighting it to the organizations in the system. We have also suggested that it may be unusual, though not unique, in the extent to which it exacerbates existing social problems. Drugs are an obvious example. It was known in the

21. Terry, "Panel Report."
22. See Tobis, *The New York City Foster Care System, 1979–1988*.
23. Lambert, "AIDS Legacy."

first year of the epidemic that HIV was associated with drug injection and blood, but for years organizations focused on countering the sexual-transmission route. Serious attention to IVDUs began about 1985, four years into the epidemic, but did not become significant until about 1987, when the rate of increase of infection among gay men leveled off.

But AIDS as a disease had more in store for New York City than infecting the large majority of IVDUs. In the same critical period the mounting social problems of the city were compounded by a new agent of social disorganization—smokable cocaine, or crack. Smokable cocaine had been around for years but it had not found its most valuable market niche—the poor minority community. Cocaine smoking probably started in the nonpoor population, perhaps most particularly in the upper and middle classes, though no one knows for sure. Marketing of the drug took place in the ghettos and the slums, as always, for that is where impoverished citizens will take the risks of arrest and drug warfare. Middle-class citizens also "deal," but not openly and on the large scale that the poor find possible. For example, Long Island suburbanites make weekly trips to the slums of New York City either to visit shooting galleries and crack houses or to buy the drugs and return home with them. In late 1989 news stories appeared saying that experts were estimating that half the crack users were nonpoor whites. Although drug abuse in general had dropped among the nonpoor, crack cocaine use had increased sharply in 1988 and 1989, as was announced in headlines like "Crack, Bane of Inner City, Is Now Gripping Suburbs."[24] But most of the deals are made in the city, and the dealers, with their small part of the huge sums made in this risky business, are tempted to partake themselves. Probably the small dealers, at the desperate edge of society, are most vulnerable to acquiring a habit.

Crack is cheap; a hit can cost from four to ten dollars. The demand for

24. Malcolm, "Crack, Bane of Inner City, Is Now Gripping Suburbs." Though this *New York Times* article is reasonably cautious, one should be aware of exaggerated claims regarding crack in the media. As far as we know, there is no strong evidence that it is instantly addictive, particularly associated with violence (incidents of violence may have nothing to do with the drug itself, but with the context and the participants), or spreading rapidly in the middle class.

cocaine, which is easily processed into crack, has risen fast, but the supply too has risen and cocaine now costs about one-tenth what it cost when the AIDS epidemic was first identified. Besides being cheap, crack is easy to try and to use. Worse still, it may be more addictive (though not instantly so) than most other major forms of substance abuse—far more than alcohol or tranquilizers. It also appears to affect women more seriously than men; they have a higher addiction rate. What's more, it can be combined with heroin to prolong the intense high,[25] and children of ten or younger who sell crack on the street have learned to sprinkle it on marijuana cigarettes to get the proper effect—otherwise it is too strong for such young bodies. All in all, it is a remarkably menacing substance. (There will be worse ones coming, including totally synthetic drugs easily made at home.)

We believe that it was the market for crack in the ghettos that resulted in its sharp rise in popularity, though it was probably the market in the more affluent areas that got the market started. It is almost as if our cities were waiting for something like crack to fill the niche of despair and poverty.

Crack users quickly encountered AIDS. In 1987 stories appeared of long sexual binges in crack houses where women sold their bodies in order to buy the drug. IVDUs were a part of this scene, and half or more of them were seropositive. The sexual activity, it now appears, is so prolonged and varied because crack stimulates sexual desire but makes it hard to reach a climax. Meanwhile, syphilis was increasing dramatically among minority groups, while it continued its decline in the majority population. (It had risen in the gay male population but fell off dramatically once precautions were taken to avoid AIDS, which, of course, are the same precautions for avoiding all sexually transmitted diseases.) In New York City the infection rate has doubled in two years. Syphilis and other sexually transmitted diseases, such as chancroid and herpes, multiplied the risk of contracting AIDS fivefold, according to one estimate. With these STDs rising, and women having prolonged sexual bouts with infected IVDUs in the crack houses, and in turn infecting non-

25. Marriott, "Latest Drug of Choice."

IVDU males, the niche for AIDS was expanded. (The infection rate for prostitutes is low, but their sexual encounters follow a different pattern. Women using crack are less likely to insist on condom use and may be more likely to have anal sex, and their partners are more likely to be IVDUs.)[26] For the first time the devastation of the non-homosexual and the non-IVDU population—heterosexual males and females and their offspring—began to resemble the pattern in Africa. There, a migratory labor population and the prostitution that accompanies it produced an epidemic of AIDS that involved neither homosexuals, anal intercourse, nor drug abuse. This pattern may be replicated in the major cities of the United States.

The consequences of crack are multiple, as the evident from New York City shows. The homicide rate has risen; in the past about 20 percent of murders were drug related, in 1988 it was at least 38 percent of the 1,867 murders in New York City involved drug dealing. The number of cocaine addicts went from an estimated 182,000 in 1986 to 600,000 in 1988. The number of parents abusing their children has tripled, from 2,627 in 1986 to 8,521 in 1988. The increase appears to be crack related; in 1985 only 11 percent of the deaths of abused children resulted from parents' drug abuse; the percent in 1987 was 73. Crack probably accounts for most of the rise in the prison population, from 10,000 to 18,000. The hospital overload is unmanageable: patients have been found free-basing cocaine in their beds, foraying into the streets to buy crack, and assaulting psychiatrists and other staff.[27] Even parental authority is further eroded: as children, recruited by local dealers, bring large sums of money (for a ghetto family) into the family, power shifts from the old to the young.[28]

The campaign against crack has been no more effective than measures against AIDS and other social catastrophes facing New York City. In 1986 Mayor Koch promised ten buildings for drug-treatment pro-

26. Kerr, "Crack and Resurgence of Syphilis Spreading AIDS."
27. Marriott, "After 3 Years, Crack Plague in New York Only Gets Worse"; French, "Crack Filling New York Hospitals."
28. Kolata, "Grim Seeds of Park Rampage."

grams, but as of February 1989 only one was in use. Two burned, two others have been condemned and require renovation, and five turned out to have liens on them. City officials said that given the paperwork involved, the whole process had gone about as smoothly as could be expected! Less than 1,000 addicts would be served.[29] At least neighborhood resistance was not a problem here; most were in fully deteriorated areas. But when the ADAPT program tried to move its administrative headquarters and its staff of eight, most of whom were black or Hispanic women, to a tree-lined neighborhood of Brooklyn brownstones, it was repeatedly vandalized (the lawn littered with condoms, the windows of its rented van broken, its burglar alarm repeatedly set off). Proposed treatment centers have been blocked in Harlem and in Queens.[30]

Nor have the schools welcomed education programs on drugs. More than two years after federal funds were made available to improve education about illegal drugs, the New York City Board of Education still had not applied for its share. The city was about to miss the deadline at the time of the news story, and the money would be lost forever—for the usual, incredible reasons: the state never gave the city the application form; it was hard to coordinate individual applications from all the local school districts, et cetera, et cetera. A total of $5.7 million was involved. New York City was the only major city in the country to delay almost three years.

New York State fared somewhat better in another federal antidrug program; it actually applied for and spent some money. Ten states, including large states with drug problems such as New Jersey and Ohio, had not applied for the current year, and eleven states, including California, New Jersey, and Maryland, had not spent the previous year's grants, which would revert. A total of $777,000 in federal funds was not being spent. At least half of the money was to be used for treatment programs for IVDUs, at least 20 percent for prevention, and 10 percent for programs for women. One of the reasons many states failed to request funds or to spend funds received was that they had no programs in these areas —hard to believe in the case of California and New Jersey. The other

29. Lee, "Paperwork, Daunting Repairs Stall '86 Plan."
30. Marriott, "Drug Program Angers Many Residents."

major reason was that the paperwork did not get done, despite prodding from the federal government.[31] Drug programs, even if they do not involve needle exchange or free needles, appear to be difficult to establish in our society, even when the money is available. Like AIDS programs, efforts to curtail drug use are stymied by public disapproval of certain behaviors, along with the familiar problems of bureaucracy and perhaps a simple lack of caring. But note that red tape is not a problem when federal funds are available for corrupt uses. In the HUD housing scandal, the "bureaucrats" in business, government, and politics proved to be very inventive. As of the fall of 1989 some 600 indictments were pending for fraud and abuse of funds in the HUD.

THE COST OF LIVING WITH AIDS

Entrepreneurship will always flourish if there is money to be made. The pharmaceutical company Burroughs-Wellcome, given exclusive rights to market a drug that government scientists developed, azidothymidine, or AZT, set the price of the drug at $8,000–$10,000 a year per patient; at the time it was the most expensive drug ever marketed. The company cited "research and development" costs (though government labs did the research), but under the National Institutes of Health licensing agreement, it did not have to document those costs. In December 1987, it cut the price by 20 percent. The federal government pays most of the cost of the prescriptions: it spent $50 million in the first six months after AZT became available, and it will spend a projected $2.4 billion by 1992 (a low projection, probably, because at the time it was not known that the drug would help those having few or no symptoms; the discovery that it would, of course, increased the demand for the drug). The company earned nearly $200 million in the first two years of production and sales, serving only 20,000 paying patients. A major investment house predicts that Burroughs will have a 40 percent earnings growth for the period 1987–1990, partly because of the rise in AZT sales.[32] The AIDS virus becomes more resistant to AZT as time

31. Tolchin, "States Not Using U.S. Antidrug Money."
32. Erdman, "AIDS Drugs."

goes on,[33] and this could limit sales, but the market is huge nevertheless: as many as 1.5 million Americans are thought to be infected, and thus eventually could use the drug. Burroughs-Wellcome will not disclose the contribution AZT is making to its rising profits, but its monopoly could overwhelm the health sector in New York City, if more "whelming" were needed. The reason for this bleak prediction is yet another irony of this remarkable epidemic, the cost of living with AIDS.

When the announcement was made that AZT was effective on those who tested positive but had no or few symptoms, the director of the National Cancer Institute declared, "This is a breakthrough, and I don't use those words often."[34] The news could mean that the estimated 400,000 of those who have the virus and a reduced number of immune system cells could postpone the development of symptoms by taking a relatively low dosage of the drug. (Another million or so who do not have reduced immunity could also benefit.) The reduced dosage would cost about $3,500 a year at today's monopoly pricing. If the price does not decline with lower recommended dosage, it might decline with competition. But any equally effective drug would be priced at near the same level; drug prices decline sharply only when the patents run out, and Burroughs-Wellcome's has a long time to run.

A recent article in the *Journal of the American Medical Association* estimates that the midrange costs of early medical intervention in asymptomatic patients to slow the progression of the disease would amount to $9,600 per person per year, of which $7,000 would be for drugs (assuming full dosage) and the rest for physician visits, serological monitoring, and counseling. In New York City perhaps 165,000 could benefit from this treatment today. At $9,600 per person that is over $1.5 billion per year for the drug and the monitoring, most of it paid for by the government, in a city where an announcement by the mayor to "seek" $40 million more for AIDS makes headlines.[35] Richard Burzon, a scientist

33. Marx, "Drug-Resistant Strains of AIDS Virus Found."
34. Hilts, "Drug Said to Help AIDS Cases."
35. Arno et al., "Economic and Policy Implications of Early Intervention in HIV Disease."

at the Institute of Medicine in the National Academy of Sciences, who has monitored AIDS costs, said, "Clearly what's going to happen, and this is very sad, is that the health care system will simply be overwhelmed, especially in a place like New York."[36] Panel after panel has said, in the words of just one, "We have an epidemic that's pushing our health-care system over the edge."[37]

Given the stigma attached to AIDS, one wonders if it is reasonable to expect society, or, rather, the elite power brokers in a city like New York, to attempt to keep 200,000 stigmatized people alive at a cost of $1 billion or more per year, year after year, as newly infected people replace those who die of other causes, well into the next century. The indifference that has been extended to AIDS and other pressing social problems in the past is staggering; would this new "burden" be shouldered?

It is possible that the drug company (and others that will be producing similar drugs) could be forced to sell at cost plus 10 percent, since the U.S. government paid for the research and since large profits have already been made on a case load of only 20,000 in 1988. But Burroughs is a British company, a country that is just as devoted to the principles of free enterprise as the United States is. Both Britain and the company would resist government interference in its pricing policy.

Irony pervades not just the supply of the drug, but the demand as well. Suppose that an alternative drug is developed by government researchers, and through special legislation the current law is held not to apply, and production and marketing rights are given to a drug company that agrees to accept only the 20 percent profit that pharmaceuticals normally make. Suppose that the cost of the drug is now only $500 per year, plus only $200 in monitoring costs because of its increased effectiveness. New York City might be able to handle this cost of $140 million a year, with substantial federal help for a decade or so, until both a vaccine and a means of giving it to those at risk become available.

What, then, about the behavior of PWAs? Under the threat of imminent death, some, at least, have moderated their risky behavior. If the

36. Shilts, *And the Band Played On.*
37. Lambert, "New York AIDS Report."

risk of the behavior can be minimized by taking the equivalent of an insulin pill, the behavior need not be moderated. Bathhouses, shooting galleries, and crack houses would be safe again. The mayor of New York might have a hard time asking taxpayers and the federal government for the money to allow those whose behavior offends to continue their offense. This is another example of how the unique nature of AIDS deflects organizational goals, undermines mandates, erodes legitimacy, and weakens the web of organizations that presumably should serve to ease inequality, poverty, and unhappiness in society.

As usual, those organizations responsible for formulating public policy and those responsible for carrying it out have been years behind in the AIDS epidemic. So much was known about blood, about the need for education, about the need for hospital beds and alternative facilities, and about the possibilities of a public backlash, but in every case systems designed to keep organizations responsive and to achieve organizational goals broke down on an unprecedented basis. The implications of keeping alive, at enormous expense, the present number of seropositive citizens, not to mention those who may be infected in the near future, make the troubles of the first few years of the epidemic look benign by comparison. It is a tragic irony that controlling the disease and extending life and health to those infected may destroy the health care and public health systems. Perhaps it is time we give serious consideration to a national health service?

A MODEL PROGRAM

Devastating epidemics usually offer few saving graces. In the case of AIDS there are two. The intensive scientific work on retroviruses may serve us in good stead when the next epidemic appears. Far less certain is the possibility that AIDS will provide the impetus, occasion, and urgency we seem to need to rebuild our social structure in such a way that epidemics have less fertile ground in which to grow. The society we have built is all too vulnerable to the onslaught of AIDS—our lack of sexual tolerance encourages furtive and anonymous practices that foster the spread of sexually transmitted diseases and discourages open disclosure and handling of the disease, and our poor urban areas are characterized by the kind of decay that encourages drug abuse, produces homelessness and prostitution, and harbors a minority community structure that cannot easily fight the disintegration it faces. Perhaps we can use the epidemic to address these issues, though little in our experience offers much hope.

One thing is certain: whatever failings there have been in organizational response to the crisis, we have not lacked for recommendations. The presidential commission formed by Ronald Reagan produced a surprisingly vigorous, inclusive set of suggestions that even addressed the problems of poverty the president did so much to exacerbate, as well as issues of civil rights for gay men, which appear to have eroded in the moral crusades of the 1980s. We would be more than happy to see the commission's recommendations vigorously pursued, but they were conspicuously ignored by President Reagan and have hardly been embraced by President Bush. That has been the fate of the commissions, panels, and the studies that Congress has ordered from its agencies, and of the numerous public and private groups that focused on New York City.

One good reason for ignoring the sweeping recommendations made is awareness of the huge cost of providing education, treatment, and care. Billions of dollars will be required to do even a minimal job, perhaps ten times the present expenditures. (The U.S. government claims to have spent about $790 million on AIDS in fiscal year 1988; New York City's agencies spent about $218 million the same year, of which $133 million were financed with city taxes, the rest with federal or state contributions. These figures were only about one-fourth the total expenditure on AIDS by all sources, private and public.) To address the social issues that allow the epidemic to continue—poverty, homelessness, crime, and drug abuse—would require another tenfold increase. The returns from these expenditures for AIDS and for social programs would be enough to delight any business executive or conservative economist. The returns from AIDS education should be an enormous savings in future health care costs; antidiscrimination campaigns will promote a more rational allocation of labor; investment in hospices and visiting nursing facilities will save on expensive hospital beds; rehabilitating vacant housing will save hospital beds and also cut down on infection rates. Money invested in social programs would decrease the cost of crime, welfare dependency, mental illness, and other problems. If the number of premature births was reduced (in part by reducing the number of teenage births), and if minority women had prenatal care and could give their children decent food and homes without lead paint, we would have far fewer mentally and physically impaired persons among the poor. If education was then improved, the present shortage of skilled and semi-skilled labor in many of our cities would disappear, and welfare expenditures would drop. And so on. Poverty is expensive; so is discrimination.

But none of the commissions studying the AIDS problem has been willing to recommend a "crash" program, a "war," a "crusade." The risks and wastes that will accompany an all-out effort will be substantial.

For example, a vigorous education program that includes instructions on cleaning needles and using condoms may well encourage a very small number of people to try drugs or extramarital sex who otherwise might have abstained. Persuading those who sell drugs to include bleach packets or provide free, non-reusable needles would require collaboration with the underworld. (No panel to our knowledge has recommended this, of course.) Legalizing drugs is increasingly discussed as a way of reducing crime and gaining access to addicts; it obviously might substantially increase the amount of addiction, perhaps most notably among the middle and upper classes. (Presumably, a sizable number of affluent, white addicts on the scene would encourage the development of far more effective rehabilitation programs, but one hesitates to suggest a gentrification of the drug-abusing population to drum up interest in upgrading rehabilitation programs.) Legalizing same-sex marriages would probably save many gay men, at least those who would choose stable pairings if they were accepted, from infection—how many it is impossible to estimate. This would not be a very risky maneuver, though it might provoke an anti-gay backlash and it would certainly complicate many civil matters regarding property, pensions, welfare benefits, and so on.

A major risk of any comprehensive program in these or any other areas is that inefficiency, waste, and corruption will taint the effort. For example, funds might be provided for, say, forty neighborhood centers in the South Bronx, each one free to dispense grants of money as well as education and the usual run of welfare services. At present a proposal of this kind would be unthinkable. The AIDS Institute would point out that the South Bronx does not have the qualified personnel (accountants and such) to administer funds and programs; existing groups would not have submitted any plans or proposals or received instructions on how to do so at meetings in the World Trade Center; favoritism and nepotism could be rife; the underworld might infiltrate the centers; and the city's housing department could never get the liens, titles, and building codes together for the centers to occupy abandoned buildings unless bribes were offered. The local politicians, it would surely be pointed out, would require "a piece of the action" before the centers could open—perhaps control over hiring, control over location, consultancy fees, speaking fees, or just plain graft.

Furthermore, there is no proven, scientifically demonstrated technique for changing the offending behaviors. The centers would be trying out dozens of ideas without undertaking controlled studies, as the National Institutes of Health and numerous AIDS experts from the social sciences would point out. The charlatans would have a field day.

Finally, a proposal of this magnitude would require an almost evangelical commitment on the part of everyone involved. Are we prepared to begin the revitalization of the South Bronx with prayer meetings each morning and sermons from the local clergy or the mayor of New York? And what will we do about the burnouts? Should they be given a generous grant and a year off to study something?

We do in fact recommend exactly this sort of initiative. What's more, what we have described has already been tried, and *it has succeeded.* A broad, inclusive, even "scattershot" approach in our slums could create jobs that the residents could fill, rehabilitate the stock of housing and eliminate homelessness, reduce chemical dependency, reduce teenage pregnancies and increase the marriage rate, spread the wealth of this nation a bit more equally, and, of course, stop AIDS.

The precedent to which we refer was the Polaris missile program, glowingly described and well documented in a book by political scientist Harvey Sapolsky of Harvard, *The Polaris System Development*.[38] It was a skirmish in the holy war against godless Communism in the 1950s, and no risks were too great. The Polaris-class submarine was to have the first submarine-launched nuclear-tipped ballistic missile. The ships would patrol as close to the Russian coast as submarines could get, ready to hit targets far inland. No one had ever built a launching system that would fire a missile from a submarine, preferably from below the surface, and we had no submarines large enough to accommodate a few missiles.

The program to do what no one had done before was sold to the nation, to the contractors, and to the navy personnel involved as a crusade. The danger of Communist invasion was less imminent and less predictable than the danger of AIDS, but forces enlisted to combat the threat were invested with a religious fervor. Daily briefings started with prayer meetings, and the wives of personnel were urged to sacrifice their home life for the safety of the country. Funds were to be ample; no part of the program could suffer because of lack of money. Congress caught the spirit too, twice voting hundreds of millions more in funds than President Eisenhower's White House asked for. Military contractors, Sapolsky noted, were able to satisfy longstanding "wish lists" for equipment and projects that were unrelated to the program. This was not called corruption or favoritism. The technology was uncertain; no existing programs had been proven efficient. Therefore eleven different launching systems were worked on at once, and the redundant ones were simply abandoned when a decision was made. No one complained of inefficiency. If underwater launches could not be achieved, surface launches would be sufficient—the goals were realistic even if the passionate desired. If a component failed a test, no inquiry was made into the reason for the failure; that would delay progress. Instead, contracts

38. Harvey M. Sapolsky, *The Polaris System Development*, quotes that follow from pages 159, 189, and 245. The conservative position that Sapolsky takes on many social issues makes his conclusions about government intervention even more convincing.

were let for alternative designs of the component, and each design was tried until one worked.

"The Polaris system traveled first class and lived first class. . . . The grade and rank structure was unusually high." Not only contractors but "the participating Navy organizations satisfied many a long-denied need from the [program] coffers." The system cost $10 billion in 1950 dollars, the cost of putting a person on the moon. The academic community relaxed its standards of objectivity, detachment, and scientific relevance, and it prospered. "The tendency was to fund any research on any remotely relevant topic that a scientist might suggest, but to keep this work completely separate from the main development effort. Some of the technical branches in the Special Projects Office had contingency funds for this purpose although they were not officially acknowledged as such." Spare parts and excess equipment abounded; waste was not a relevant concept. Contracts were distributed widely throughout the nation to build support should commitment to the crusade wane. The program was pronounced a great success; it is one of the most famous successes in the military build-up of the cold war. Its cost was astronomical by the standards of the day, but rarely questioned.

The contrasts with AIDS and poverty are clear. We demand precise accounting from grass-roots groups with dying people on their hands; we resist giving money to inexperienced people and untried community agencies; we worry about paying as much as $25,000 for New York City program directors and fear the misuse of agency funds; we are afraid to fund duplicate efforts or experimental programs, so we wait for techniques that are effective and efficient; we won't settle for incremental behavioral changes but insist on total abstinence, even though protective measures of varying degrees would save lives; we are cautious in social science research because our knowledge is limited; we rely on whatever personnel is available in poorly funded state, city, and local agencies rather than going first-class to attract the best talent; and we cannot get our national or local leaders to declare a holy war on poverty and AIDS, but only on nonmarital sex and intravenous drug use, and in this way we limit our weapons against death itself. There is no legitimate excuse for not trying the Polaris model.

BIBLIOGRAPHY

"Administration Faulted on Homeless Aid Program." *New York Times,* October 2, 1988.

AIDS Surveillance Unit, New York City Department of Health. *AIDS Surveillance Update.* November 29, 1989.

Altman, Denis. *AIDS in the Mind of America.* Garden City, N.Y.: Anchor Press, 1986.

Altman, Lawrence K. "As Hepatitis B Spreads, Physicians Reconsider Vaccination Strategy." *New York Times,* August 1, 1989.

——— "U.S. to Ease Methadone Rules in Bid to Curb AIDS in Addicts." *New York Times,* March 3, 1989.

Andrulis, Dennis P., Virginia Beers Weslowski, and Larry S. Gage. "The 1987 U.S. Hospital AIDS Survey." *Journal of the American Medical Association* 262 (August 11, 1989): 784–794.

Arno, Peter S., and Robert G. Hughes. "Local Policy Responses to the AIDS Epidemic: New York and San Francisco." *New York State Journal of Medicine,* 87 (May 1987): 264–272.

Arno, Peter S., et al. "Economic and Policy Implications of Early Intervention in HIV Disease." *Journal of the American Medical Association,* 262 (September 15, 1989): 1493–1498.

Barron, James. "Health Chief Sees Obstacle to AIDS Needle Plan." *New York Times,* March 15, 1988.

Bay Area Reporter, July 14, 1988; June 2, 1988; September 15, 1988; October 15, 1988; November 17, 1988; and December 8, 1988.

Bayer, Ronald. *Private Acts, Social Consequences: AIDS and the Politics of Public Health*. New York: Free Press, 1989.

Becker, Marshall H., and Jill G. Joseph. "AIDS and Behavioral Change to Reduce Risk: A Review." *American Journal of Public Health*, 78 (April 1988): 394–410.

Berg, Ellen. "The AIDS Experience." *ASA Footnotes*, December 1988.

Bigel Institute. *New York City's Hospital Occupancy Crisis*. Mimeo. The Bigel Institute at Brandeis University and the United Hospital Fund of New York, 1988.

Bishop, Katherine. "Gap between Cost of Drug Epidemic and State Money Shuts California Clinic." *New York Times*, February 3, 1989.

"Black Men in St. Louis Slain at Highest Rate, Study Says." *New York Times*, August 3, 1989.

Blattner, William A. "A Novelistic History of the AIDS Epidemic Demeans Both Investigators and Patients." *Scientific American*, 258 (October 1988): 148–151.

Blendon, Robert J., and Karen Donelan. "Discrimination against People with AIDS." *New England Journal of Medicine*, 319 (October 13, 1988): 1022–1026.

Boffey, Philip M. "Homeless Plight Angers Scientists." *New York Times*, September 20, 1988.

——— "Research Group Says AIDS Cases May Be Twice the U.S. Estimate." *New York Times*, August 20, 1988.

——— "Tests of a Potential Drug for AIDS Beginning after Months of Delay." *New York Times*, July 24, 1988.

Bowles, Samuel, David M. Gordon, and Thomas E. Weisskopf. *Beyond the Wasteland: A Democratic Alternative to Economic Decline*. Garden City, N.Y.: Doubleday, Anchor Press, 1983.

Brandt, Allan M. *No Magic Bullet: A Social History of Venereal Disease in the United States since 1880*, expanded edition. New York: Oxford University Press, 1988.

Carbine, M. E., and P. Lee. *AIDS into the 90's: Strategies for an Integrated Response to the AIDS Epidemic*. Washington, D.C.: National AIDS Network, 1988.

Carter, Zoe. "Local Hero: ADAPT and Survive." *New York Magazine*, May 9, 1988, p. 35.

"Casual Drug Use Is Sharply Down." *New York Times*, August 1, 1989.

Centers for Disease Control. *HIV / AIDS Surveillance Report*. December 1989.

————*Mortality and Morbidity Weekly Report*, 37, no. SS-3 (July 1988): 4-6.

Chira, Susan. "Cuomo Says State Will Step Up AIDS Research and Assist Victims." *New York Times*, June 23, 1983.

Colby, David C., and David G. Baker. "State Policy Responses to the AIDS Epidemic." *Publius, The Journal of Federalism*, 18 (Summer 1988): 113–123.

Congressional Record, May 25, 1983, pp. H3341–3344.

Conrad, Peter. "The Social Meaning of AIDS." *Social Policy*, 17 (Summer 1986): 51–65.

"Council Calls for End to Free-Needles Plan." *New York Times*, December 7, 1988.

Crawford, Mark. "Superconductor Funds Flat." *Science*, 239 (March 4, 1988): 1089, and 239 (August 7, 1987): 593.

Crewdson, John. "The Great AIDS Quest." *Chicago Tribune*, Special Report, November 19, 1989.

Culliton, Barbara J. "Legion Fever: Postmortem on an Investigation That Failed." *Science*, 194 (December 3, 1976): 1025–1027.

Des Jarlais, Don C., Cathy Casirel, and Samuel Friedman. "The New Death among IV Drug Users. In *AIDS: Principles, Practices, and Politics*, ed. Inga B. Corless and Mary Pittman-Lindeman, pp. 135–150. Washington, D.C.: Hemisphere Publishing Corp., 1988.

Des Jarlais, Don C., Samuel R. Friedman, and David Strug. "AIDS and Needle Sharing within the IV-Drug Use Subculture." In *The Social Dimensions of AIDS: Method and Theory*, ed. Douglas A. Geldman and Thomas M. Johnson, pp. 111–125. New York: Praeger, 1986.

Dicker, Frederick, and Ann Bollinger. "Top Narc Takes Shot at AIDS Needle Plan." *New York Post*, February 2, 1988.

Dunne, Richard. "New York City: Gay Men's Health Crisis." In *AIDS: Public Policy Dimensions*, ed. John Griggs. pp. 155–169. New York: United Hospital Fund of New York, 1987.

Dutton, Diane. *Worse Than the Disease: Pitfalls of Medical Progress*. New York: Cambridge University Press, 1988.

Erdman, Karen. "AIDS Drugs." *Public Citizen*, May–June 1989, pp. 10–16.

Evans, Heidi, and Mike Santangelo. "O'C Blasts Addict Plan." *New York Daily News*, February 1, 1988.

Fineberg, Harvey V. "The Social Dimensions of AIDS." *Scientific American*, 258 (October 1988): 128–134.

Fitzgerald, Frances. *Cities on a Hill: A Journey through Contemporary*

American Cultures. New York: Simon and Schuster, 1986.

"Forecasts of AIDS Fall Short, U.S. Study Says." *New York Times*, June 26, 1989.

Foundation Center. *AIDS Funding: A Guide to Giving by Foundations and Charitable Organizations.* New York: Foundation Center, November 1988.

Fox, Daniel M. "AIDS and the American Health Polity: The History and Prospects of a Crisis of Authority." *Milbank Quarterly*, 64, suppl. 1 (1986): 7–33. Reprinted in *AIDS: The Burdens of History*, ed. Elizabeth Fee and Daniel M. Fox, pp. 316–343. Berkeley: University of California Press, 1988.

Fox, Daniel M., Patricia Day, and Rudolf Klein. "The Power of Professionalism: Policies for AIDS in Britain, Sweden, and the United States." *Daedalus*, 118 (Spring 1989): 93–112.

French, Howard W. "Again, Debate Over Private Hospitals' Public Duty." *New York Times*, March 9, 1989.

———"Crack Filling New York Hospitals with Frustration, Fear and Crime." *New York Times*, May 10, 1989.

———"Hospitals Overwhelmed as Poor in New York City Search for Care." *New York Times*, December 4, 1988.

———"In Brooklyn, a Hospital Faces Its Own Mortality." *New York Times*, March 20, 1989.

———"New York Health Care Failure Charged." *New York Times*, December 8, 1988.

———"Unlikely Coalition Fights Cut Proposed in Medicaid Budget." *New York Times*, February 26, 1989.

Freudenberg, Nicholas. "Historical Omissions: A Critique of *And the Band Played On*." *Health / PAC Bulletin*, Spring 1988, pp. 16–20.

———"The Politics of AIDS Education." Paper presented at the First National Symposium on AIDS Prevention, Baltimore, Md., May 28, 1987.

Freudenberg, Nicholas, Jacalyn Lee, and Diana Silver. "How Minority Community Organizations Respond to the AIDS Epidemic." Paper presented at the Fourth International Conference on AIDS, Stockholm, Sweden, June 1988.

Friedman, Samuel R., and Cathy Casriel. "Drug Users' Organizations and AIDS Policy." *AIDS & Public Policy Journal*, 3, no. 2 (1988): 30–36.

Friedman, Samuel R., J. L. Sotheran, A. Abdul-Quader, B. J. Primm, D. Des Jarlais, P. Kleinman, C. Mauge, D. S. Goldsmith, W. El-Sadar, and R. Maslansky. "The AIDS Epidemic among Blacks and Hispanics." *Milbank*

Quarterly, 65, suppl. 2 (1987): 455–499

Gargan, Edward A. "Partisan Dispute Delays Bill to Mitigate Shoreman's Cost." *New York Times*, June 26, 1983.

General Accounting Office. *AIDS Prevention: Views on the Administration's Budget Proposals*, August 1987.

———*Coping with AIDS in the Workplace*. December 1987.

Gillman, Cherni L. "Genesis of New York City's Experimental Needle Exchange Program." *International Journal on Drug Policy*, 1 (September–October 1989): 28–32.

Green, R. "End the Cutbacks." *Village Voice*, January 14, 1986.

Gross, Jane. "Amid Bias, Homosexuals Are Finding New Understanding." *New York Times*, February 4, 1988.

———"Emergency Room: A Crack Nightmare." *New York Times*, August 6, 1989.

———"Epidemic in Urban Hospitals: Wounds from Assault Rifles." *New York Times*, February 21, 1989.

Gussow, Zachary. "Social Policy and Chronic Disease Control." In *Leprosy, Racism, and Public Health*. Boulder, Colo.: Westview Press, 1989.

Gutis, Philip S. "Attacks on U.S. Homosexuals Held Alarmingly Widespread." *New York Times*, June 8, 1989.

Harrison, Bennett, and Barry Bluestone. *The Great U-Turn: Corporate Restructuring and the Polarizing of America*. New York: Basic Books, 1988.

Hiatt, Fred. "Tainted U.S. Blood Blamed for AIDS' Spread in Japan." *Washington Post*, June 23, 1988.

Hilts, Philip. "Drug Said to Help AIDS Cases with Virus But No Symptoms." *New York Times*, August 18, 1989.

Imperato, Pascal James. "New York's Homeless." *New York State Journal of Medicine*, 87 (January 1987): 1–3.

Institute of Medicine, *The Future of Public Health*. Washington, D.C.: National Academy Press, 1988.

Interagency Task Force on AIDS. *New York City Strategic Plan for AIDS*. May 1988.

Intergovernmental Health Policy Project, George Washington University. *AIDS: A Public Health Challenge*. Vol. 1, *Assessing the Problem*. Washington, D.C.: Public Health Service, October 1987.

———"State-Only Expenditures for AIDS: Major Trends, Fiscal Years 1983–1986." *Focus On*, no. 18 (October 1987).

Johnston, David. "Radical Rehab." *New York Times*, August 13, 1989.

Jones, James H. *Bad Blood: The Tuskegee Syphilis Experiments*. New York: Free Press, 1981.

Kagay, Michael. "Poll Finds Antipathy towards AIDS Victims." *New York Times*, October 12, 1988.

Kaplan, Edward H. "Can Bad Models Suggest Good Policies? Sexual Mixing and the AIDS Epidemic." *Journal of Sex Research*, 26 (August 1989): 301–314.

———"Needles That Kill: Modeling Human Immunodeficiency Virus Transmission via Shared Drug Injection Equipment in Shooting Galleries." *Review of Infectious Diseases*, 11 (1989): 289–298.

Kaplan, Edward H., and Paul R. Abramson. "So What If the Program Ain't Perfect? A Mathematical Model of AIDS Education." *Evaluation Review*, 13 (April 1989): 107–122.

Kerr, Peter. "Crack and Resurgence of Syphilis Spreading AIDS among the Poor." *New York Times*, August 20, 1989.

———"Experts Find Fault in New AIDS Plan." *New York Times*, February 7, 1988.

———"Syphilis Surge and Crack Use Raising Fears on Spread of AIDS." *New York Times*, June 29, 1988.

Kolata, Gina. "AIDS Test May Fail to Detect Virus for Years, Study Finds." *New York Times*, June 1, 1989.

———"Congress, NIH Open Coffers for AIDS." *Science*, 221 (July 29, 1983): 436–437.

———"Grim Seeds of Park Rampage Found in East Harlem Streets." *New York Times*, May 2, 1989.

———"New York Shelters, a Last Stop for Hundreds of AIDS Patients." *New York Times*, April 4, 1988.

Krieger, N. *The Politics of AIDS*. Oakland, Calif.: Frontline Pamphlets, 1986.

Kwitny, Jonathan. "At CDC's AIDS Lab: Egos, Power, Politics and Lost Experiments." *Wall Street Journal*, December 12, 1986.

Lambert, Bruce. "AIDS Drives Jobs Away, Study Says." *New York Times*, March 7, 1989.

———"AIDS Legacy: A Growing Generation of Orphans." *New York Times*, July 17, 1989.

———"AIDS Patients Seen Straining Hospitals." *New York Times*, March 3, 1989.

———"AIDS Services: A Disjointed Network." *New York Times*, May 5,

1989.

———"Black Clergy Set to Preach about AIDS." *New York Times*, June 10, 1989.

———"Concentration of AIDS Cases Posing Serious Problem for Some Hospitals." *New York Times*, August 11, 1989.

———"Cuomo Sets AIDS Plan, Admitting It Falls Short." *New York Times*, February 16, 1989.

———"Debate Swirls over Cuts in Health Agency Budgets." *New York Times*, May 31, 1988.

———"Drug Group to Offer Free Needles to Combat AIDS in New York City." *New York Times*, January 8, 1988.

———"Ethics and Needles." *New York Times*, August 13, 1988.

———"Flaws in Health Care System Emerge as Epidemic Rages." *New York Times*, February 8, 1989.

———"Halving of Estimate on AIDS Is Raising Doubts in New York." *New York Times*, July 20, 1988.

———"Hospital Shortages Hurt Patient Care in New York." *New York Times*, March 22, 1988.

———"Koch's Record on AIDS: Fighting a Battle without a Precedent." *New York Times*, August 27, 1989.

———"Koch to Seek $40 Million More for AIDS." *New York Times*, May 15, 1989.

———"New York AIDS Report Assails Inadequate Financing." *New York Times*, August 1, 1989.

———"Outlook Dim for Expanding Health Care." *New York Times*, April 5, 1988.

———"Puzzling Questions Are Raised on Statistics on AIDS Epidemic." *New York Times*, July 22, 1988.

———"State AIDS Council Attacks Cuomo over Delays." *New York Times*, March 5, 1989.

———"Study Finds Alarming AIDS Rate in Homeless Shelter." *New York Times*, June 5, 1989.

Laumann, E. O., et al. "Monitoring the AIDS Epidemic in the United States: A Network Approach." *Science*, 244 (June 9, 1989): 1186–1189.

Lee, Felicia R. "Paperwork, Daunting Repairs Stall '86 Plan for Drug Centers," *New York Times*, February 3, 1989.

Lee, Philip R., and Peter S. Arno. "AIDS and Health Policy." In *AIDS: Public Policy Dimensions*, ed. John Griggs, pp. 3–20. New York: United Hospital

Fund of New York, 1987.

Linebarger, Charles. "Scandal at Shanti." *San Francisco Magazine*, October 1988, pp. 66–69.

——— "Scandal Surfaces at the Shanti Project; But Why Was It Kept Secret for So Long?" Unpublished manuscript.

London, Herbert. "Free Needles? Brace Yourselves for the Inevitable Lawsuits and Scandals." *New York Post*, February 2, 1988.

Lyall, Sarah. "Hospital Calls Layoff of 300 a Last Resort." *New York Times*, February 6, 1989.

Mahar, Maggie. "Pitiless Scourge; Separating Out the Hype from Hope on AIDS." *Barron's*, March 13, 1989, pp. 6–7, 16–27.

Malcolm, Andrew. "Crack, Bane of Inner City, Is Now Gripping Suburbs." *New York Times*, October 1, 1989.

Malinowsky, H. Robert, and Gerald J. Perry, eds. *AIDS Information Sourcebook, 1988–1989*, 2d ed. Phoenix, Ariz.: Oryx Press, 1989.

Marmor, Theodore R. "American Medical Policy and the 'Crisis' of the Welfare State: A Comparative Perspective." *Journal of Health Politics, Policy and Law*, 11, no. 4 (1986): 617–631.

Marriott, Michel. "After 3 Years, Crack Plague in New York Only Gets Worse." *New York Times*, February 20, 1989.

——— "Drug Program Angers Many Residents of Boerum Hill." *New York Times*, July 2, 1989.

——— "Koch Picks 8 Sites in 3 Boroughs to House Homeless AIDS Patients." *New York Times*, October 31, 1988.

——— "Latest Drug of Choice for Abusers Brings New Generation to Heroin." *New York Times*, July 13, 1989.

——— "Needle Exchange Angers Many Minorities." *New York Times*, November 7, 1988.

——— "New York Alters Needle Plan to Combat AIDS." *New York Times*, January 30, 1989.

Marx, Jean. "Drug-Resistant Strains of AIDS Virus Found." *Science*, 243 (March 24, 1989): 1551–1552.

Massey, Douglas S., and Nancy A. Denton. "Hypersegregation in U.S. Metropolitan Areas: Black and Hispanic Segregation along Five Dimensions." *Demography*, 26 (August 1989): 373–391.

May, Clifford D. "Hospitals Take Budget Woes to Congress." *New York Times*, March 6, 1989.

May, Robert M., and R. M. Anderson. "Transmission Dynamics of HIV Infection." *Nature*, 326 (March 12, 1987): 137–142.

Mays, V. M., and S. D. Cochran. "Acquired Immunodeficiency Syndrome and Black Americans: Special Psychosocial Issues." *Public Health Reports,* 102, no. 2 (1987): 224–231.

McFadden, Robert. "Health Department Closes Down Gay Cinema." *New York Times,* October 1, 1988.

——— "Koch Criticized on Plan to Open AIDS Shelters." *New York Times,* November 1, 1988.

McNeill, William H. *Plagues and Peoples.* Garden City, N.Y.: Doubleday, Anchor Press, 1976.

National Public Radio. "All Things Considered" (radio broadcast), July 24, 1988.

Newfield, Jack, and Wayne Barrett. *City for Sale: Ed Koch and the Betrayal of New York.* New York: Harper and Row, 1989.

New York State Comptroller. "Projected Cost of the Treatment of Acquired Immune Deficiency Syndrome." Mimeo, Report 11-88, July 8, 1987.

O'Connor, John Cardinal, and Mayor Edward I. Koch. *His Eminence and Hizzoner: A Candid Exchange.* New York: Morrow, 1989.

Office of Technology Assessment. *How Effective Is AIDS Education?* Staff Paper No. 3. Washington, D.C.: Office of Technology Assessment, June 1988.

———*Review of the Public Health Service's Response to AIDS: A Technical Memorandum.* February 1985.

Okun, Stacey. "Lack of Nurses Impedes New York AIDS Care." *New York Times,* February 23, 1988.

Oppenheimer, Gerald M. "In the Eye of the Storm: The Epidemiological Construction of AIDS." In *AIDS: The Burdens of History,* ed. Elizabeth Fee and Daniel M. Fox, pp. 267–300. Berkeley: University of California Press, 1988.

Paine, Leslie H. W., ed. *Health Care in Big Cities.* New York: St. Martin's, 1978.

Panem, Sandra. *The AIDS Bureaucracy.* Cambridge, Mass.: Harvard University Press, 1988.

Perrow, Charles. *Complex Organizations: A Critical Essay,* 3d ed. New York: Random House, 1986.

———"Demystifying Organizations." In *The Management of Human Services,* ed. Rosemary Sarri and Yeheskel Hasenfeld, pp. 105–120. New York: Columbia University Press, 1978.

———*Normal Accidents: Living with High Risk Technologies.* New York: Basic Books, 1984.

————"A Society of Organizations." Mimeo, Yale University, 1989.

Philadephia Commission on AIDS. *Report to the Community*. 1988.

Pindyck, Johanna. "AIDS and the Blood Service System." In *AIDS: Public Policy Dimensions*, ed. John Griggs, pp. 85–100. New York: United Hospital Fund, 1987.

Piore, Nora, Purlaine Lieberman, and James Linnane. "Public Expenditures and Private Control? Health Care Dilemmas in New York City." *Milbank Memorial Fund Quarterly*, 55 (Winter 1977): 79–116.

Pomrinse, S. David, George B. Allen, and John C. Rossman. "Health Care in a Big City in a Time of Fiscal Crisis." In *Health Care in Big Cities*, ed. Leslie H. W. Paine, pp. 282–292. New York: St. Martin's, 1978.

Rabin, Judith A. "The AIDS Epidemic and Gay Bathhouses: A Constitutional Analysis." *Journal of Health Politics, Policy and Law*, 10 (Winter 1986): 729–747.

Renshaw, Vernon, Edward A. Trott, Jr., and Howard L. Friedenberg. "Gross State Product by Industry, 1963–1986." *Survey of Current Business*, 68 (May 1988): 30–46.

"Realism on AIDS" (editorial). *Nation*, February 13, 1988.

Report of the Presidential Commission on the Human Immunodeficiency Virus Epidemic. Washington, D.C.: Government Printing Office, June 24, 1988.

Richwald, Gary A., Donal E. Morisky, Garland R. Kyle, Alan R. Kristal, Michele M. Gerber, and Joan M. Friedland. "Sexual Activities in Bathhouses in Los Angeles County: Implications for AIDS Prevention Education." *Journal of Sex Research*, 25 (May 1988): 169–180.

Rimer, Sara. "Lawsuit Seeks Drug Treatment on Demand." *New York Times*, June 14, 1989.

Risman, Barbara, and Pepper Schwartz. "Sociological Research on Male and Female Homosexuality." *Annual Review of Sociology*, 14 (1988): 125–147.

Robohm, Amy M. "AIDS: The Impact on Black and Hispanic Communities." Mimeo, Yale University Department of Sociology, December 1988.

Rosenthal, Michell S. "Methadone Clone: A Bad Quick Fix." *New York Times*, July 1, 1989.

Rossman, John C., and S. David Pomrinse. "New York City." In *Health Care in Big Cities*, ed. Leslie H. W. Paine, pp. 50–79. New York: St. Martin's, 1978.

Ryan, Michael. "Give People Hope, Not Drugs." *Daily News Parade*, September 25, 1988.

Sapolsky, Harvey M. *The Polaris System Development: Bureaucratic and*

Programmatic Success in Government. Cambridge, Mass.: Harvard University Press, 1972.

Schieber, George J. *Financing and Delivering Health Care: A Comparative Study of OECD Countries.* Paris: OECD, 1987.

Senak, Mark S. "The Lesbian and Gay Community." In *Aids and the Law: A Guide for the Public*, ed. Harlon L. Dalton and Scott Burris, pp. 290–300. New Haven: Yale University Press, 1987.

Shilts, Randy M. *And the Band Played On: Politics, People, and the AIDS Epidemic.* New York: St. Martin's, 1987.

Shulman, Lawrence C., and Joanne E. Mantell. "The AIDS Crisis: A United States Health Care Perspective." *Social Science and Medicine*, 26, no. 10 (1988): 979–988.

Siegel, Marc. "The Wall-to-Wall Emergency at City Hospitals." *New York Times*, August 12, 1989.

Smith, Jeanne, and Sergio Piomelli. "The War on AIDS." *New York Times*, January 22, 1989.

Sontag, Susan. *AIDS and Its Metaphors.* New York: Farrar, Straus and Giroux, 1989.

"Study Finds Antibodies for AIDS in 1 in 61 Babies in New York City." *New York Times*, January 13, 1988.

Sullivan, Ronald. "Experts Testify AIDS Epidemic Strikes the City." *New York Times*, May 17, 1983.

——— "Parishioners Block Archdiocese's AIDS Shelter." *New York Times*, August 31, 1985.

Swanstrom, Todd. "Homeless: A Product of Policy." *New York Times*, March 23, 1989.

Terry, Don. "Panel Report Finds New York City Is Failing Its Sickest Poor Children." *New York Times*, July 25, 1989.

Thurow, Lester C. "A Surge in Inequality." *Scientific American*, 256 (May 1987): 30–37.

Tobis, David Michael. *The New York City Foster Care System, 1979–1988: The Rise and Fall of Reform.* Ph.D. diss., Yale University, 1989.

Tolchin, Martin. "States Not Using U.S. Antidrug Money." *New York Times*, April 17, 1989.

Turner, Charles F., Heather G. Miller, and Lincoln E. Moses, eds. *AIDS: Sexual Behavior and Intravenous Drug Use.* Washington, D.C.: National Academy Press, 1989.

Verhovek, Sam Howe. "Cuomo Is Being Fought on Medicaid Cuts." *New York*

Times, February 24, 1989.

Waite, Thomas. "New York Shuts 2 Gay Theatres as AIDS Threats." *New York Times*, February 12, 1989.

Waterman, Daniel. "Tracks of the Disease." *New Journal* (Yale University), December 4, 1987.

Weinberg, David S., and Henry W. Murray. "Coping with AIDS: The Special Problems of New York City." *New England Journal of Medicine*, 317 (December 3, 1987): 1469–1473.

Weiss, Robin, and Samuel O. Thier. "HIV Testing Is the Answer—What's the Question?" *New England Journal of Medicine*, 319 (October 13, 1988): 1010–1012.

Williams, Lena. "Inner City under Siege: Fighting AIDS in Newark." *New York Times*, February 6, 1989.

Williamson, Jeffrey G., and Peter H. Lindert. *American Inequality: A Macroeconomic History*. New York: Academic Press, 1980.

Wilson, William Julius. *The Truly Disadvantaged: The Inner City, the Underclass, and Public Policy*. Chicago: University of Chicago Press, 1987.

Winkelstein, W., D. M. Lyman, N. S. Padian, R. Grant, M. Samuel, J. A. Wiley, R. E. Anderson, W. Lang, J. Riggs, and J. A. Levy. "Sexual Practices and Risk of Infection by the AIDS-Associated Retrovirus: The San Francisco Men's Health Study." *Journal of the American Medical Association*, 257 (1987): 321–325.

INDEX

Abyssinian Baptist Church, Harlem, 100, 125
Acquired Immune Deficiency Syndrome (AIDS): cases of, 2, 55–57, 95–96, 104; compared with other damaging conditions and behaviors, 55–67; consequences of, 63–64; costs of, 12–13, 64–67, 175–79; cultural tolerance of persons with, 58–59; as epidemic, 3–4, 11–17, 64–67; as gay men's disease, 11, 15, 74–75, 102; medical aspects of, 63–64; medicalization of, 7–8, 82–83; moralization of, 7–8; as plague, 9; research on, 23–25; as self-inflicted disease, 6,7, 9, 57–59; as result of "sinful behavior," 99–100; as unique, 3–5, 55–67, 149–51. *See also* Human Immunodeficiency Virus, transmission of; Newborns, with AIDS
ACT UP (AIDS Coalition to Unleash Power), 109
ADAPT (Association for Drug Abuse Prevention and Treatment), 84–85, 101, 107, 109, 117–26, 133, 136, 169, 174
Africa, AIDS in, 12, 15
AIDS Emergency Fund, 116n
AIDS Institute. *See* New York State AIDS Institute
AIDS Project New Haven (APNH), 113
AIDS Resource Center, 135
Altman, Denis, 20
American Academy of Pediatrics, 16
American Association of Blood Banks, 42, 43n
American Foundation for AIDS Research (AmFAR), 29
American Red Cross, 39, 42, 87, 110, 110n
Andrulis, Dennis P., 137n
Austria, AIDS in, 7
Axelrod, David, 30, 82–83, 122, 123